MIND DIET
INSTANT POT C

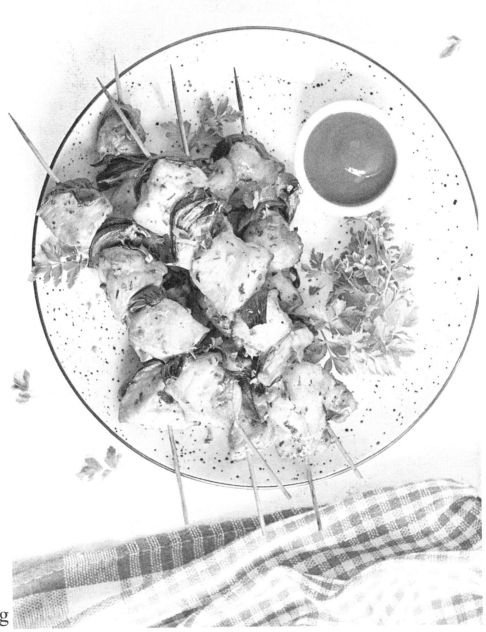

Henry Irving

TEXT COPYRIGHT © HENRY IRVING

LEGAL & DISCLAIMER

The information contained in this book and its contents is not designed to replace or take the place of any form of medical or professional advice; and is not meant to replace the need for independent medical, financial, legal, or other professional advice or services, as may be required. The content and information in this book has been provided for educational and entertainment purposes only.

The content and information contained in this book has been compiled from sources deemed reliable, and it is accurate to the best of the Author's knowledge, information, and belief. However, the Author cannot guarantee its accuracy and validity and cannot be held liable for any errors and/or omissions. Further, changes are periodically made to this book as and when needed. Where appropriate and/or necessary, you must consult a professional (including but not limited to your doctor, attorney, financial advisor, or such other professional advisor) before using any of the suggested remedies, techniques, or information in this book.

Upon using the contents and information contained in this book, you agree to hold harmless the Author from and against any damages, costs, and expenses, including any legal fees potentially resulting from the application of any of the information provided by this book. This disclaimer applies to any loss, damages or injury caused by the use and application, whether directly or indirectly, of any advice or information presented, whether for breach of contract, tort, negligence, personal injury, criminal intent, or under any other cause of action. You agree to accept all risks of using the information presented inside this book.

You agree that by continuing to read this book, where appropriate and/or necessary, you shall consult a professional (including but not limited to your doctor, attorney, or financial advisor or such other advisor as needed) before using any of the suggested remedies, techniques, or information in this book.

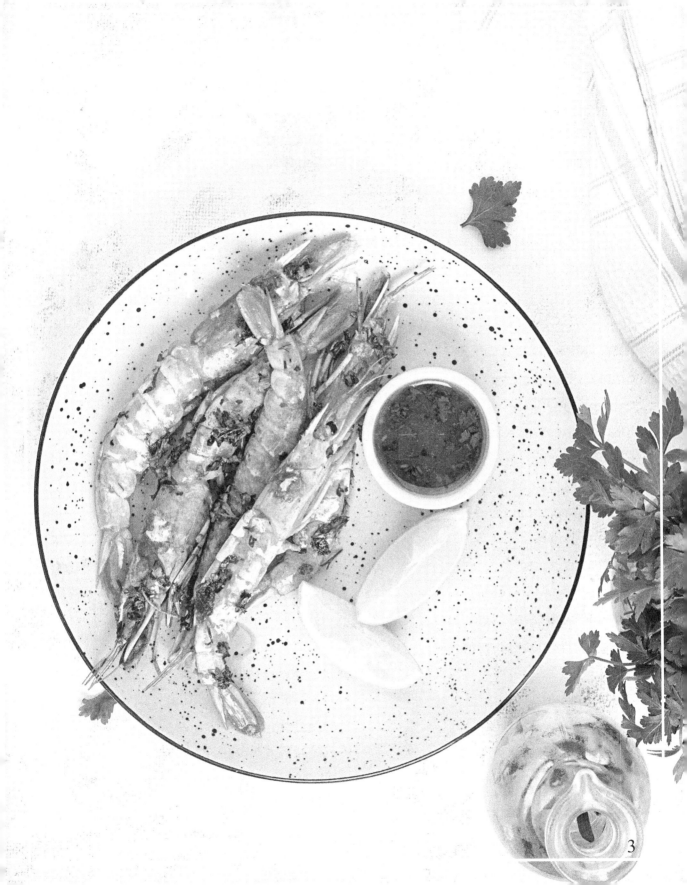

TABLE OF CONTENT

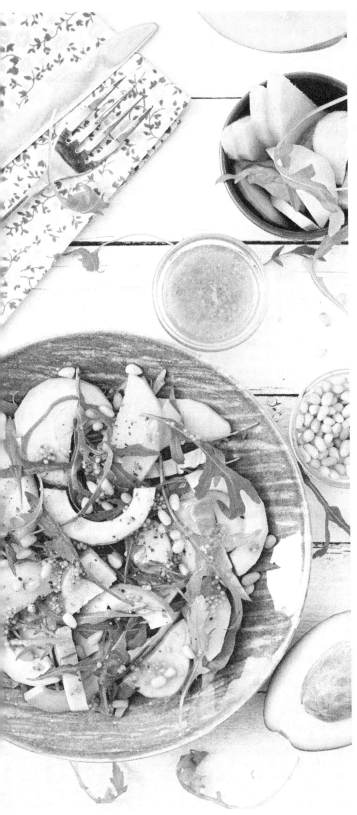

DESCRIPTION

Dementia and Alzheimer's are something we've all heard about. At first, you forget what kind of ice cream you ate in the park yesterday and whether you turned off the gas when you left the house. Subsequently, illness takes away more and more valuable and important parts of life: birthdays of loved ones, names, and faces of loved ones.

The biggest misconception people have is that they think it's typical for older people that it's normal for them to forget things. But it all works a little differently.

Alzheimer's disease is the most common form of dementia, which is a disorder of the brain that affects a person's life every day. It is characterized by deterioration of memory, speech, mental faculties, and other cognitive skills that affect a person's ability to live life to the fullest. Everything happens gradually, from forgetting some little things or a person's distraction. These seem to be all simple little things, but they can lead to these illnesses in the aftermath.

You cannot diagnose Alzheimer's or Dementia on your own. If you suspect that you or your family members have it (the signs are becoming more and more obvious), be sure to make an appointment with your doctor. There is no need to be afraid, there is nothing wrong with going to the doctor, on the contrary, early diagnosis and help will give you a better chance of delaying more debilitating symptoms. With the right medicine, you prolong your independence and make the most of your life.

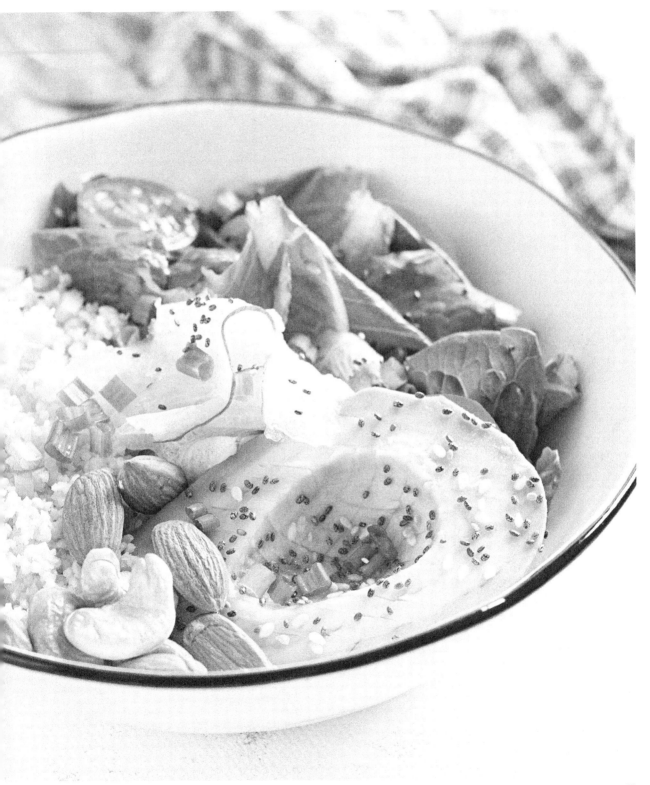

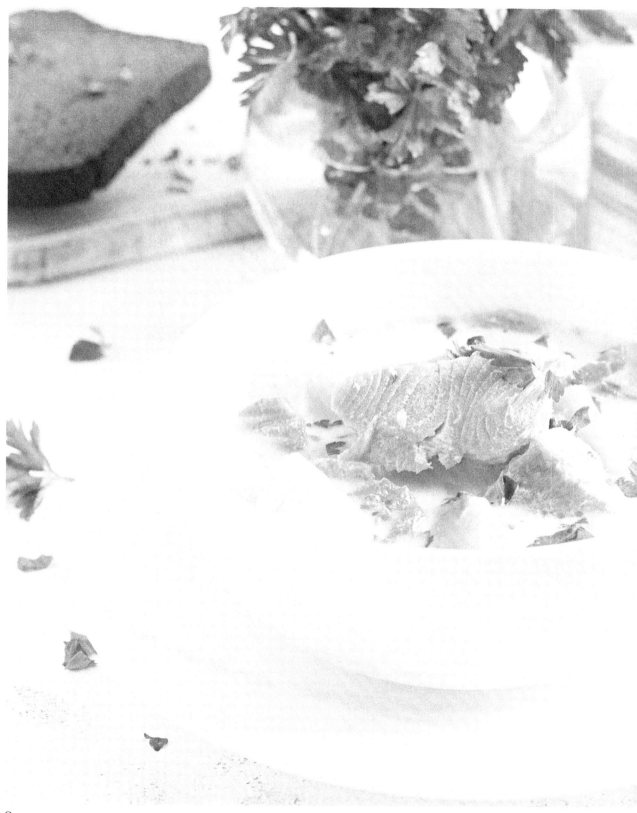

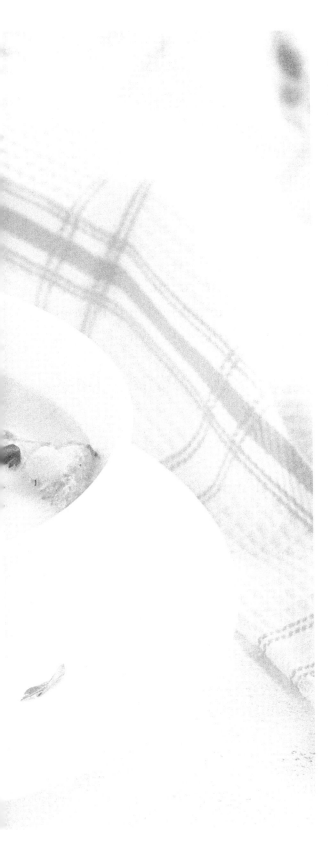

Alzheimer's disease is, unfortunately, a common disease in the elderly, but steps can be taken at any age to prevent it. First and foremost is to change your diet and lifestyle.

Many people don't realize that the foods they eat and the lifestyle they lead affect their long-term health (even if they are perfectly healthy at the moment).

This book is written specifically to introduce you to the MIND diet, which is so important for every person at every age. There are diets that are good not only for the body but also for the mind. One such is the MIND diet, whose effectiveness has been scientifically proven.

Each chapter in this book reveals the secrets of healthy living, not only for the body but also for the health of the brain. This book carefully selects important things, such as the development and diagnosis of Alzheimer's disease, and the appropriate foods that the MIND diet recommends.

The purpose of this book is to help you learn how to prevent Alzheimer's disease and dementia by changing your diet plan and lifestyle. It's never too late to change your life for the better by changing your eating habits, which may save your life later and allow you to live out your old years with peace of mind.

BENEFITS OF THE MIND DIET

Research on the influence of diet and lifestyle on the development of senile diseases, including senile dementia, is becoming increasingly popular. Whereas previously scientists usually focused on individual nutritional components, today more attention is being paid to eating behavior and habits in general.

Can brain health be improved through diet?

Nutrition not only affects the body but also brain health and mental performance. In this book, I, nutritionist Henry Irving, want to talk about how nutrition and brain health are connected and what to eat to maintain mental clarity in old age and reduce the risk of developing dementia.

Dementia is a syndrome in which memory, thinking, speech, and the ability to orient, count, cognize, and reason are degraded.

What's important to know:

Dementia affects mostly the elderly but is not considered a normal condition when a person is aging.

There are about 50 million people with dementia worldwide, and 10 million get it each year.

Alzheimer's disease is the most common cause of dementia, accounting for 60-70% of cases worldwide.

Dementia is the seventh most common cause of death from the disease and one of the leading causes of disability and addiction among the elderly.

Dementia has a physical, psychological, social, and economic impact not only on those who suffer from it, but also on their caregivers - families, and society as a whole.

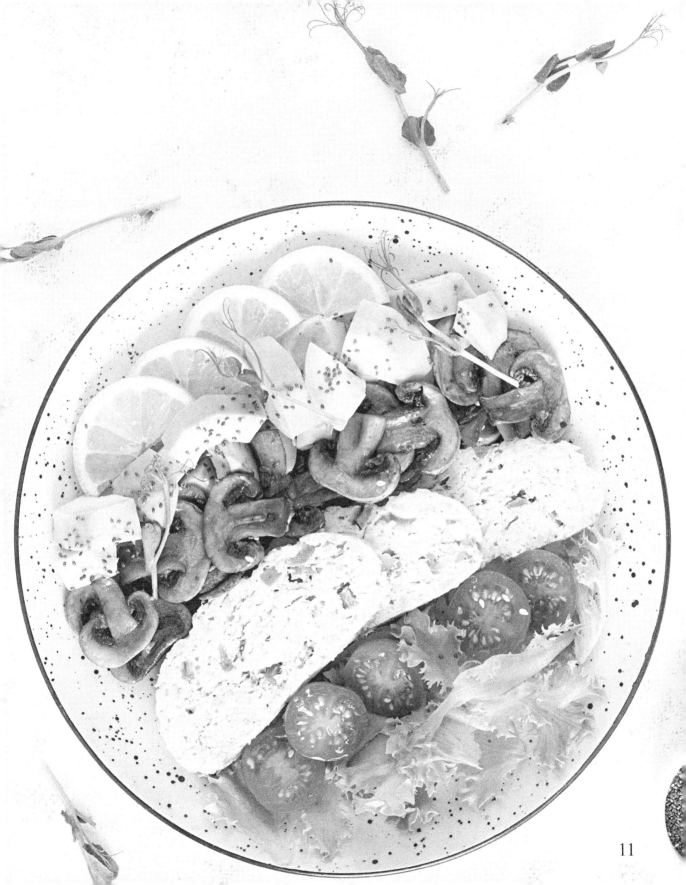

11

Why does dementia develop?

Sometimes, as a person grows older, abnormal accumulations of proteins form in his or her brain tissue. This is a sign of Alzheimer's disease, the most common form of dementia. As brain cells are affected, the number of chemical mediators that help transmit signals between neurons decreases. Over time, different parts of the brain diminish, and the area responsible for memory is the first to suffer.

It is not known exactly why abnormal protein deposition occurs. Scientists say that it begins many years before a person develops symptoms.

The main factors that increase the risk of developing Alzheimer's disease are:
  - Age is the most important factor. The likelihood of the disease doubles every 5 years after the age of 65;
  - Genes - a small percentage of the disease is linked to mutations in three genes that can be inherited;
  - Down syndrome;
  - Head injuries;
  - Cardiovascular disease;
  - Lifestyle and conditions associated with it: bad habits (smoking, heavy alcohol), obesity, diabetes, high blood pressure.

Currently, there is no therapy to cure dementia or change the course of its development. Research on numerous medications is ongoing. That's why it's especially important to work on preventing age-related brain disorders. One way is to change your eating habits.

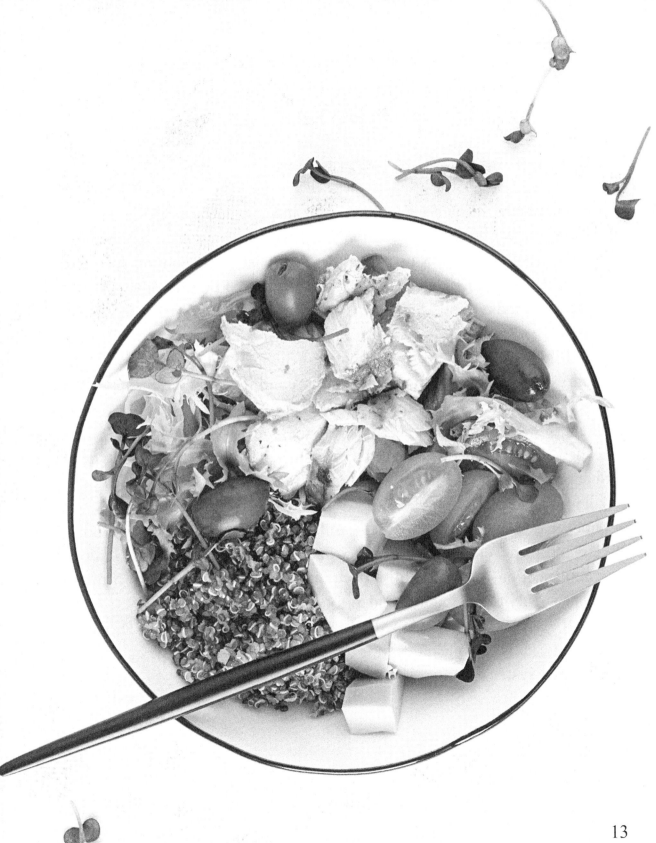

MIND diet - your way to brain health

I love the phrase, «You are what you eat,» and as a nutritionist, I attest to that. Research on the effects of nutrition on the development of senile diseases, including senile dementia or Alzheimer's disease, is becoming increasingly popular. While in the past scientists usually focused on individual nutritional components, today more attention is being paid to a person's eating behavior and habits as a whole.

Two of the diets recognized as the most beneficial for human health, DASH (Dietary Approaches to Stop Hypertension) and the Mediterranean diet, gave rise to the so-called MIND diet.

Scientists at Rush University Medical Center (Chicago) found that older people may benefit from a special MIND diet, even when they have pathogenic deposits of beta-amyloid and tau proteins (the same plaques and tangles that later cause Alzheimer's disease).

A study has shown that people who follow the MIND diet clearly reduce the likelihood of developing Alzheimer's disease by 53%. Those who follow the recommendations partially still reduce their risk by a third (35%) if their diet consists mostly of the recommended foods from the MIND diet.

The MIND diet was developed by Martha Claire Morris, M.D., of Rush University, and her colleagues. It is a hybrid of the Mediterranean diet and the DASH diet system.

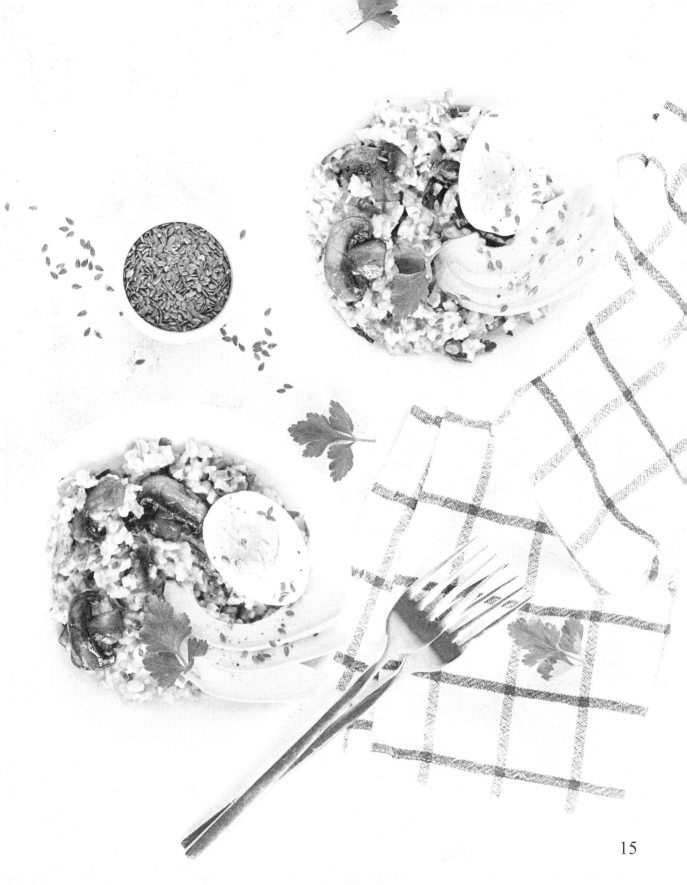

Now, let's focus briefly on the Mediterranean diet

The Mediterranean diet is more than a diet. It is a lifestyle. It's a way of eating in order to live a full and healthy life. People following the Mediterranean diet have been linked to a lower risk of Alzheimer's disease and cancer, better overall cardiovascular health, and an extended lifespan. The building blocks that comprise a Mediterranean diet are foods rich in healthy oils, low in saturated fat, and filled with vegetables and fresh fruits.

The Mediterranean diet focuses on typical foods and recipes you'd find in Mediterranean-style cooking. This diet includes consuming lots of vegetables and grains, fruits, rice, and pasta while limiting fats, replacing salt with herbs and spices, and eating fish and poultry instead of red meat. The Mediterranean diet does not contain a lot of red meat. Nuts are a part of a healthy part of this diet.

The Mediterranean diet reflects various eating habits of the countries near the Mediterranean Sea, mainly Southern Italy, Greece, Morocco, France, and Spain. Due to their unique locality, the climate supports fresh fruits, vegetables, and some of the world's best seafood. This diet isn't focused on limiting your total consumption of fat; instead, it focuses on making smarter choices about the kinds of fat you consume.

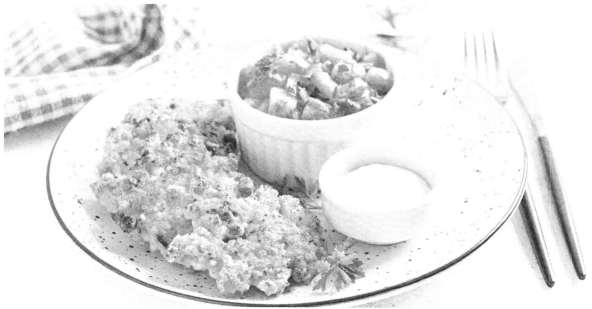

This diet discourages people from eating trans-fats and saturated fats, both of which have been linked to heart disease.

Grains used in the Mediterranean diet are preferably whole grain, which generally contains very little in the way of unhealthy trans-fat. Instead, the bread is eaten either dipped in olive oil or eaten plain. This cuts down significantly on the number of trans and saturated fats normally associated with eating bread.

Wine plays a large role in the Mediterranean diet. A glass of wine is normally included with each evening meal.

This means 5 ounces or less of wine for anyone over the age of 65 and for people under 65 no more than 10 ounces daily. If you have any history of alcohol dependency or abuse, I suggest refraining altogether from consuming alcohol as part of your diet. The same goes if you already have liver or heart disease.

Olive oil is the primary source of fat in this type of diet. It actually provides monounsaturated fat, which is the kind of fat that helps reduce the levels of LDL cholesterol when utilized instead of trans or saturated fats. The "Extra virgin" and "virgin" olive oils are considered to have undergone the least processing. They also happen to contain the largest levels of protective plant compounds responsible for providing antioxidant effects.

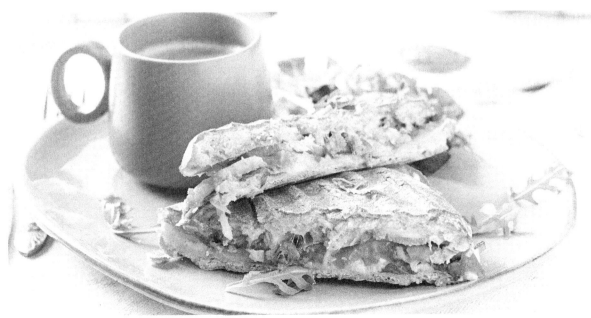

DASH diet and its secrets

The DASH diet is considered one of the healthiest meal plans for lowering blood pressure. It includes foods that are rich in potassium, calcium, and magnesium: these substances help control a person's blood pressure. All you have to do to follow this diet is to reduce your intake of unhealthy fats, refined sugar, and sodium. The basics of the diet are:

- vegetables,
- fruits,
- whole grains,
- low-fat or low-fat dairy products,
- fish,
- poultry,
- beans and nuts.

Consumption of fatty meat, fatty dairy products, coconut oil, and palm oil is limited.

The Mediterranean diet and DASH can lower blood pressure and reduce a person's risk of heart disease and diabetes.

These food systems are good at preventing cardiovascular disease, which can impair brain health at any age. However, the ratio of foods adopted in them is not one hundred percent suitable for correcting brain function. Therefore, scientists have created a hybrid of the two «best diets on the planet.

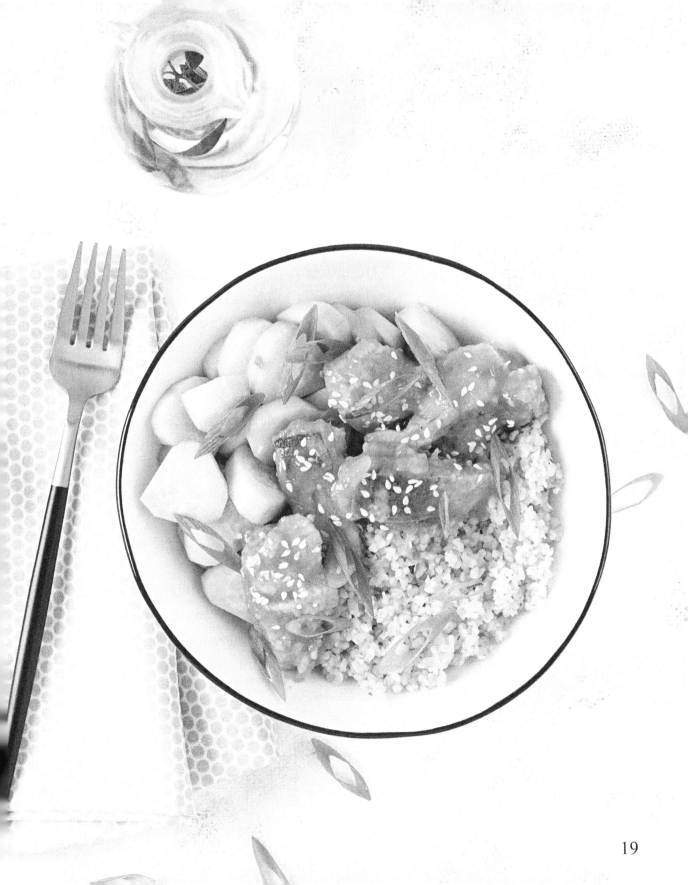

Mechanisms of action of the MIND diet

One of the key mechanisms of this diet on brain function is the reduction of oxidative stress as well as inflammatory processes. Antioxidants (found in berries and fruits) and vitamin E (found in oils, nuts, and seeds) protect the brain from free radicals. When these molecules accumulate in our bodies in large amounts, they can cause great harm. Brain cells are especially vulnerable to the effects of free radicals, which is why it is so important to combat them at any age to prevent senile dementia.

One of the main components of a person's diet is fish. It, a source of valuable omega-3 fatty acids, has an anti-inflammatory function for the human body. By reducing inflammation in the brain, we also help preserve cognitive abilities and remove the development of senile dementia.

One potential mechanism could be to reduce beta-amyloid formation, which researchers believe is a major cause of Alzheimer's disease and dementia. After all, beta-amyloids accumulate in the brain and form amyloid plaques, leading to the death of brain cells.

But remember, poor diet is only one part of developing Alzheimer's disease. Move every day, use stairs instead of elevators, and engage in structured physical activity at least twice a week. Also, control your stress levels, get plenty of sleep, connect with loved ones more often, and make your life as conscious as possible in all aspects of it.

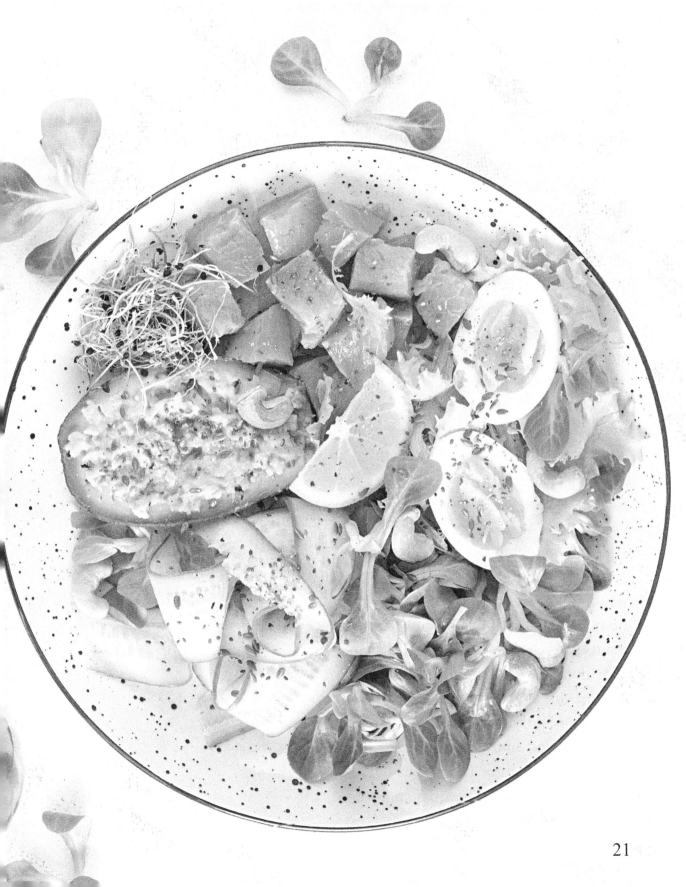

FOODS TO EAT AND AVOID

«Everything we eat directly affects our brains,» explains Priyanka Rohatgi, chief nutritionist and director of nutrition at Apollo Hospitals. «Frequent consumption of drinks high in sugar can lead to impaired memory and slow down learning. It's also best to avoid smoked foods. They contain nitrosamines, which produce fats that are toxic to brain function,» says the doctor.

In addition to sugary drinks and smoked meats, you should also minimize your consumption of cheese (no more than once a week), red meat (three times a week), fried meat (no more than once a week), and desserts and industrial cookies.

As I mentioned in the previous chapter, this diet should not be followed by people who fear the risk of getting dementia disease, but by anyone who wants to keep their brain in good shape. You don't have to be an older person to start this diet. You may be 30 or 40 years old and you can start consuming fresh berries and vegetables, reduce processed and junk foods, eat healthy fats, seafood, and minimize sugar and junk food intake.

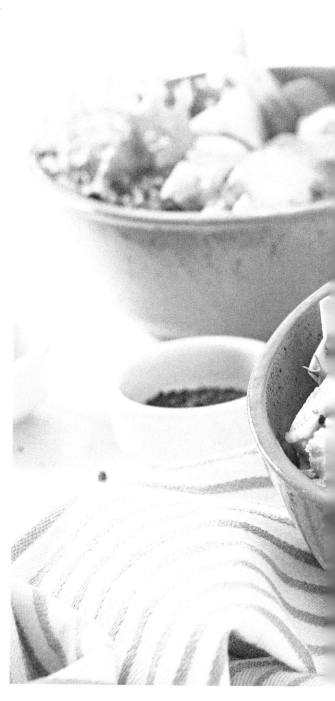

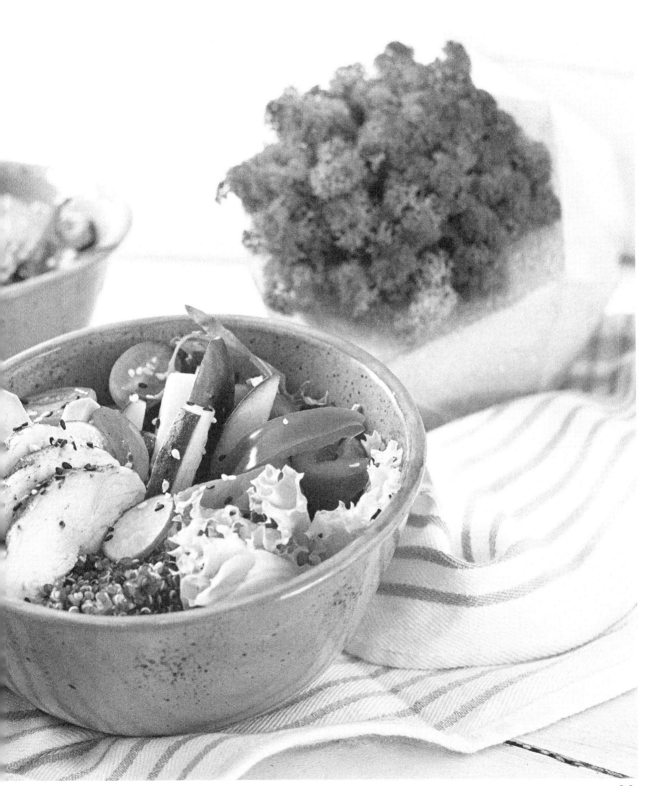

Here are the foods that are appropriate for this diet. I want to point out that you do not have to be overweight to start this diet.

Berries. Eat berries at least two servings a week. One serving is one cup. Berries are the only fruit specifically designed for the MIND diet;

Green leafy vegetables. Eat at least 1 servings a day. This includes spinach, leafy cabbage, kale, greens, endive, kohlrabi, etc.;

All other vegetables. Add at least 1 serving of other vegetables to your salad. Preferably, they should be non-starchy vegetables, because they have a high concentration of nutrients with low calories;

Nuts. Eat at least 6 servings of nuts per week. You can also add a mix of nuts to salads;

Legumes. Eat 1 serving of legumes (beans, peas, mung bean, chickpeas, lentils, soybeans) every other day;

Whole-grain foods. You should eat at least three servings a day. One serving is ½ cup of cooked product or 1 slice of bread;

Fish. Eat at least 1 serving of fish a week. Choose fatty fish as they are the source of omega-3 fatty acids.

Poultry. Eat white poultry (chicken, turkey) at least 2 servings per week. Choose lean cuts of meat;

Olive oil. Use extra virgin olive oil as the basic vegetable oil in the kitchen; it enriches your dishes with healthy fats and vitamins;

Wine. You can drink no more than one glass (140 ml) of red or white wine per day. If you enjoy a glass of wine at dinner, you may not give up this habit on the MIND diet.

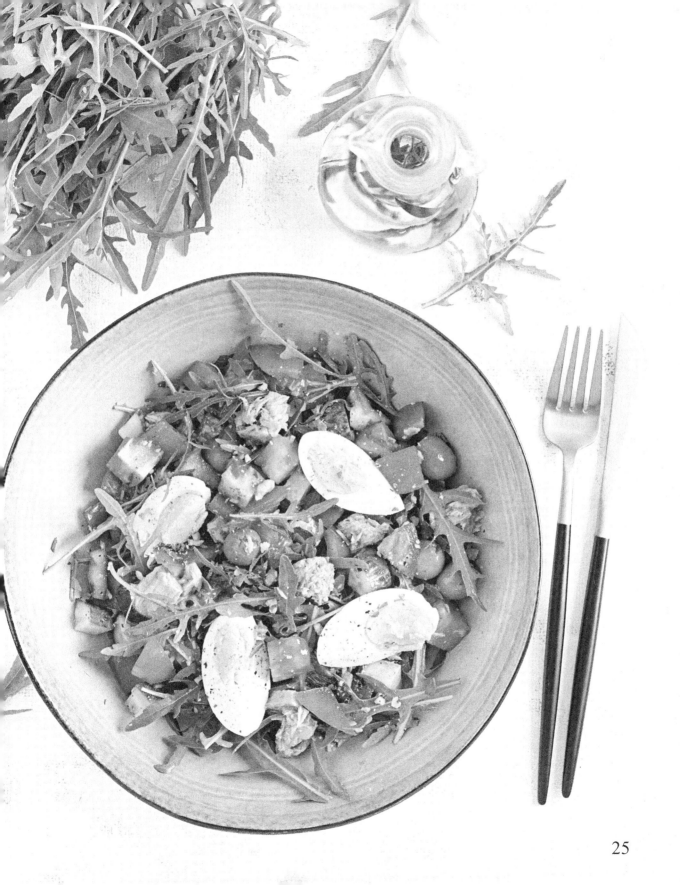

Foods to avoid on the MIND diet

Butter and margarine. Limit your butter intake to 1 tablespoon or less per day;

Red meat. Try to eat no more than 3 servings per week. This includes beef, lamb, pork, and other products based on them;

Cheese. Limit fatty cheeses to one serving per week;

Pastries and sweets. Try to limit sweets to no more than 4 treats per week;

Fried foods and fast food. No more than one meal of such food per week, or better yet, give up such food altogether.

It's pretty obvious: what we eat can affect how effectively we think. So be careful about what's on your plate!

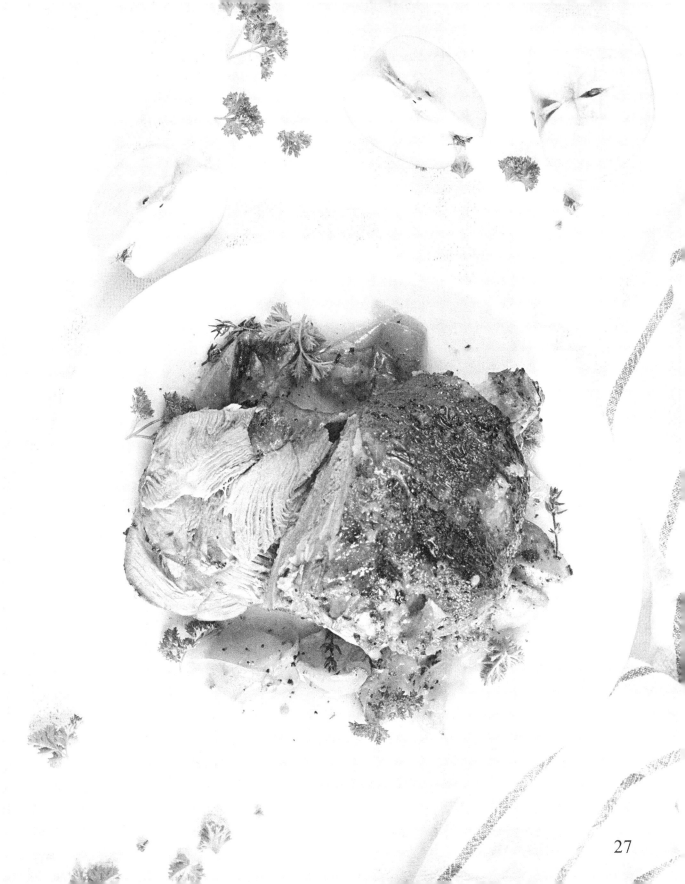

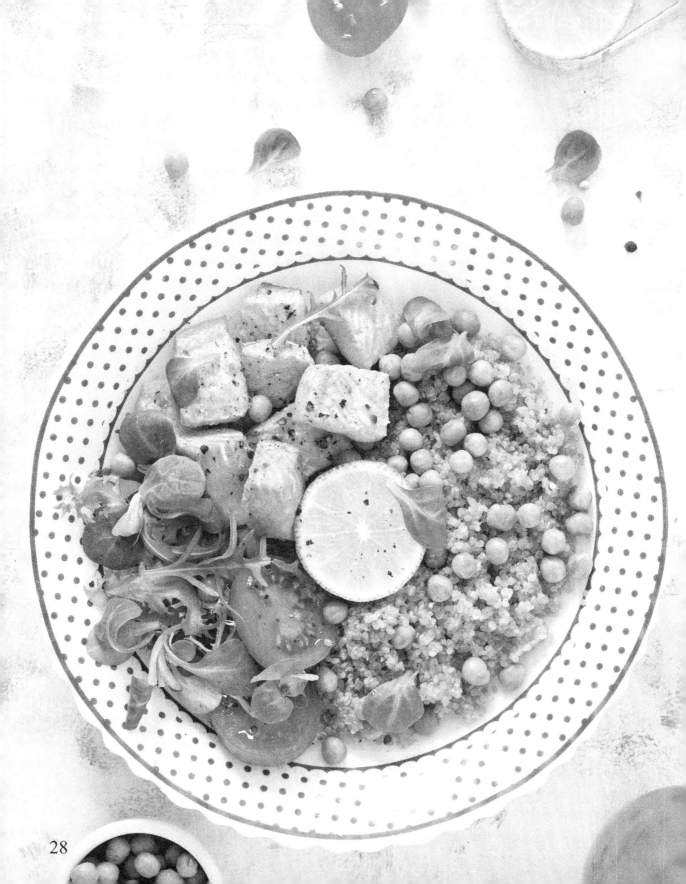

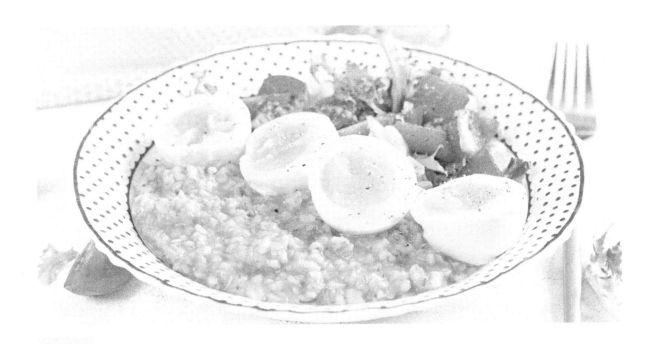

WHAT LIFESTYLE SHOULD YOU ADOPT TO REDUCE YOUR RISK OF ALZHEIMER'S

If it seems that you forget everything, and even the simplest information quickly fades from memory, you need to do something about it. What exactly, we'll tell you point by point. It's simple, the main thing is to start.

I think you understand that eating right is only the first step to your health. Improve the quality of your life and get into the right habits. These steps will help you prevent Alzheimer's and slow its deterioration.

Move every day. Walk and use stairs instead of elevators. And also control your stress levels: sleep abundantly, use meditation and relaxation techniques, and make your life as conscious as possible in all aspects of it.

You're never too old to start taking care of your brain health. The earlier you reinforce the steps mentioned above, the longer they will serve you and give you stronger support. Let's take a closer look at each of these steps.

Exercise

According to the Alzheimer's Disease Research and Prevention Foundation, frequent physical activity will reduce the risk of developing Alzheimer's disease by up to 50 percent. In addition, frequent exercise will slow further deterioration in people who have already begun to develop cognitive problems. If you're wondering how long you should exercise per week, the answer is simple - at least 150 minutes a week. The best combination is cardio and strength training. But don't be intimidated by these numbers. If you are a beginner, you can always start with simple exercises like walking or swimming. It will be very helpful to introduce coordination and balance exercises. The best balance and coordination exercises are tai chi, yoga and Pilates (use balancing balls). You may not be attracted to gyms, but you can always walk your block or ride your bike.

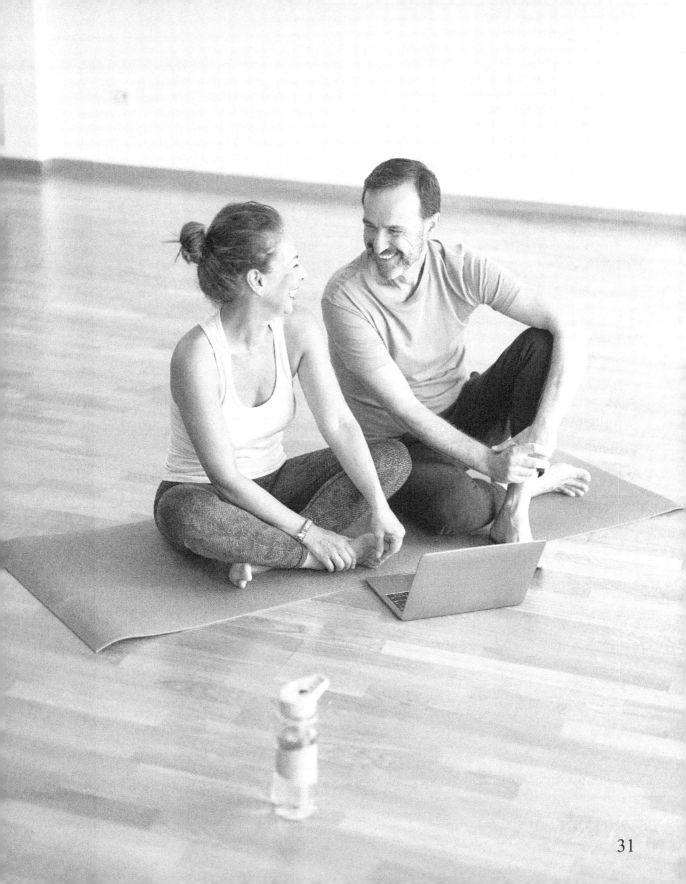

Healthy Diet

Since the diet is based mostly on fresh fruits and vegetables, healthy oils and whole grains, and lean meats and seafood, it's easy to see why this diet is considered healthy. Mix it with a glass of red wine and you have a fun and easy diet for your health. Even moderate adherence to the MIND diet is good for your brain.

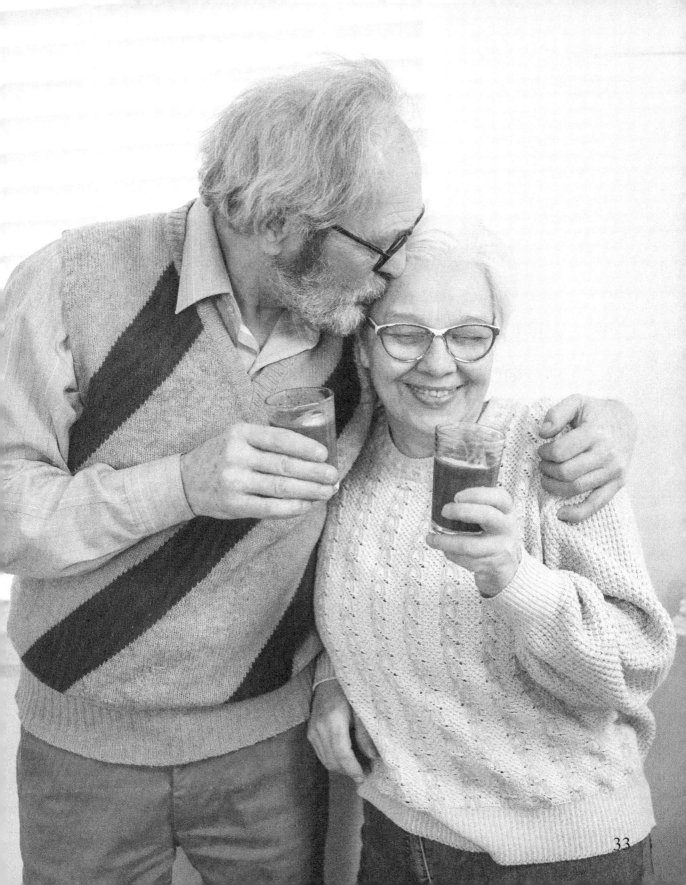

Social Activity

Keeping yourself socially active can protect you from Alzheimer's in your old age, so make time for some social interaction.

You don't have to be the soul of the party. All you need is a constant connection with your friends. Many people become isolated as they age, but new friends don't have an expiration date. You can make new friends at any age. Just go to an exhibition, go to a park or any public place where you can meet new people and just talk to them.

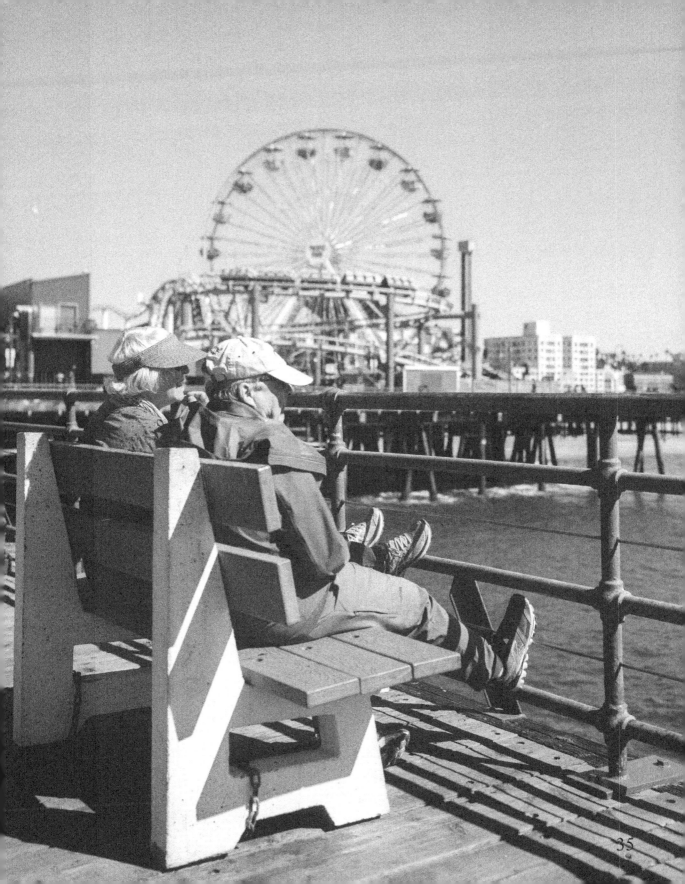

Healthy Sleep

Our body was not designed to live without proper sleep. If you've been sleep-deprived at least once in your life, you already know how it affects your thinking and cognitive performance. It affects your mood and your physical movements, and you are slower to respond. Lack of sleep can greatly affect the development of Alzheimer's disease and dementia.

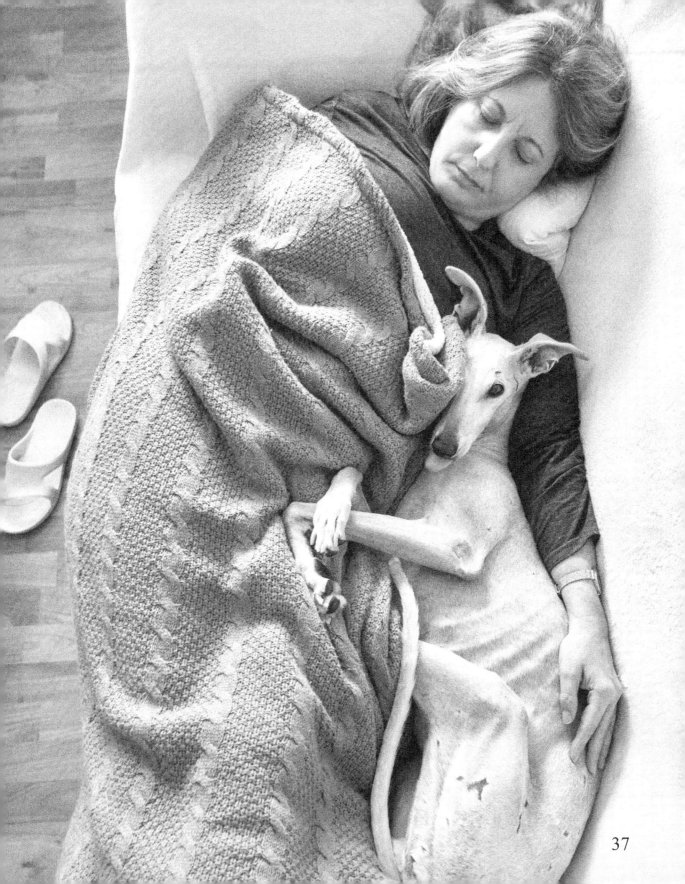

Mental Stimulation

The learning process never ends. If you stimulate your mental activity by learning new things, you will reduce your risk of developing Alzheimer's disease and dementia. Develop your intelligence. The brain becomes more efficient if we make it work harder: do crossword puzzles, learn foreign languages, memorize street names. Learning something new every day keeps your brain alert. It is also very important and useful to train your memory. Here are five easy ways to do this:

- Recall yesterday's events. You need to remember what you did the day before. For example, who you talked to or what you read.
- Read aloud. Read aloud a column from the first page of the morning paper. Do it as fast as you can and write down the time you did it in.
- Communicate. It is very important for a person to communicate with other people to keep his or her brain healthy.
- Do things with your hands. Cooking, playing a musical instrument, drawing, writing, sewing - these activities also activate the prefrontal cortex. It is very good to change the left hand to the right hand or vice versa. This way you activate the two hemispheres of the brain.
- Count in your mind. When we count in our mind, the part of the brain responsible for memory and attention starts to work.

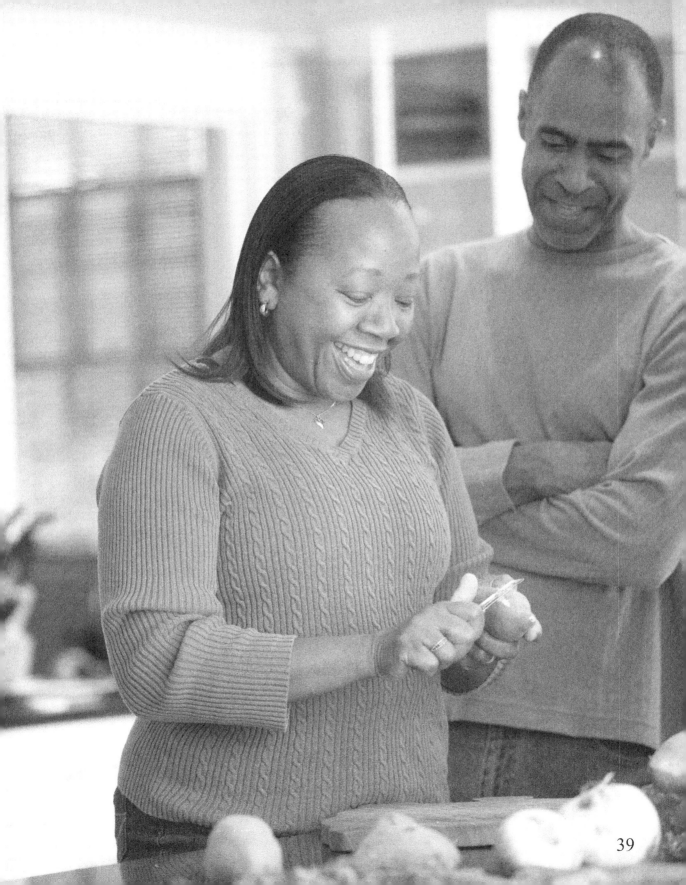

39

Enhance Your Mood

The diet can help you to be positive, even when things aren't going your way. Healthy living does that. When you have eaten enough food to fuel you with lots of nutrients, your body notices. Fulfillment and productivity enhance your mood. For one, applying the diet correctly will make you feel like you're doing something good for yourself and thus enhances your overall mood.

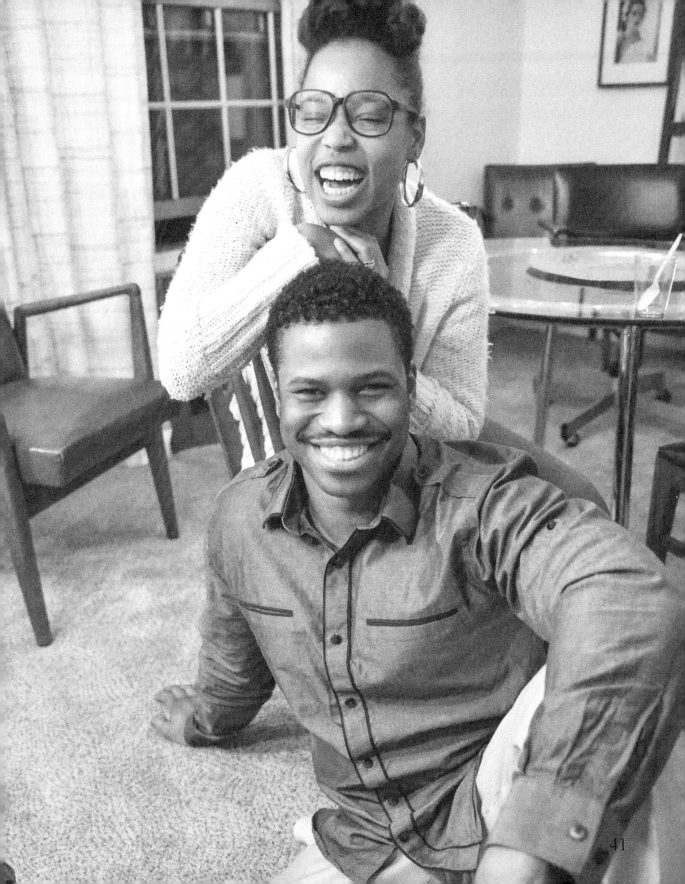

Keep Blood Pressure Under Control

Hypertension or high blood pressure is linked to a high risk of dementia. High blood pressure ruins tiny blood vessels in the parts of the brain that are responsible for cognition and memory. Start checking your blood pressure regularly. Obtain a blood pressure device and check it at home. When you hold your blood pressure on track, you can be in control of taking responsibility to support it that way. If you can't obtain such a device, create sure to schedule a doctor's appointment regularly so they can measure it for you.

Never ignore low blood pressure. Although it affects distant fewer people, low blood pressure can reduce the blood flow in your brain. The main symptoms are blurred vision, dizziness, fatigue, and unsteadiness when you stand up. Schedule a doctor's appointment if your blood pressure is constantly low.

It's not required to point out that smoking is severely damaging your health. Cutting this nasty custom is an outstanding way to reduce the risk of Alzheimer's sickness and dementia. Smokers over the age of sixty-five have almost eighty percent higher risk of this sickness compared to people who don't' smoke. Hold your lungs free of smoke and breathe deeply for a minimum of ten minutes a day.

Hold your cholesterol levels balanced. Studies propose that there may be a link between high cholesterol and the risk for Alzheimer's and dementia. This is particularly emphasized in people who have high cholesterol levels in their center age.

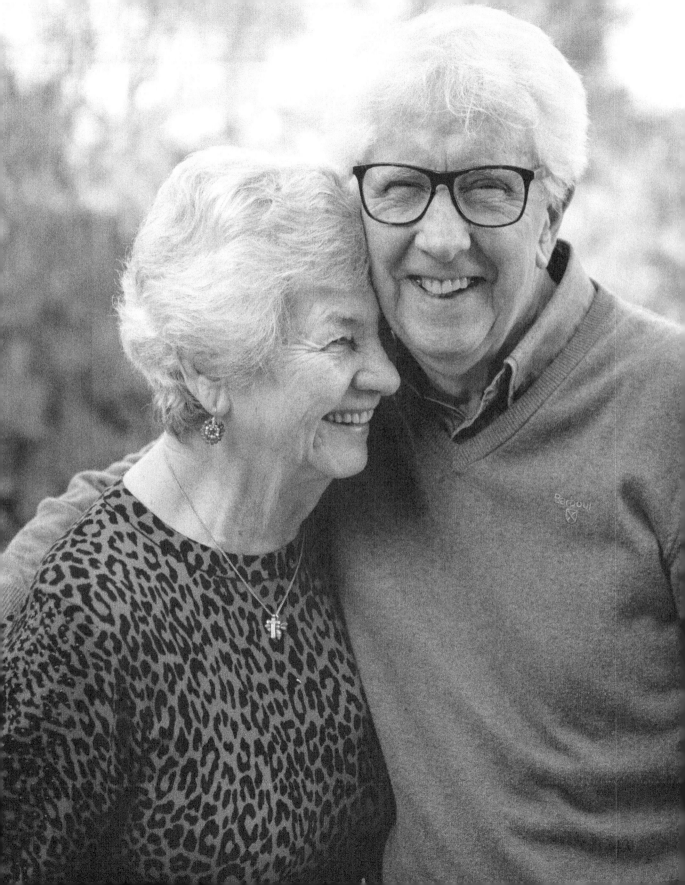

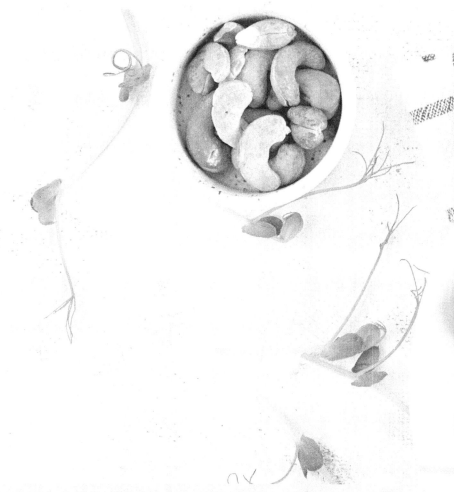

Well, all the secrets are revealed. And I think each of you understands that everything is quite simple. Make your life better, follow these great tips, switch to the MIND diet and you will feel better. I will repeat to you once again my favorite phrase «It is never too early to change your life and develop good habits that may later save your life and allow you to live your older years in peace».

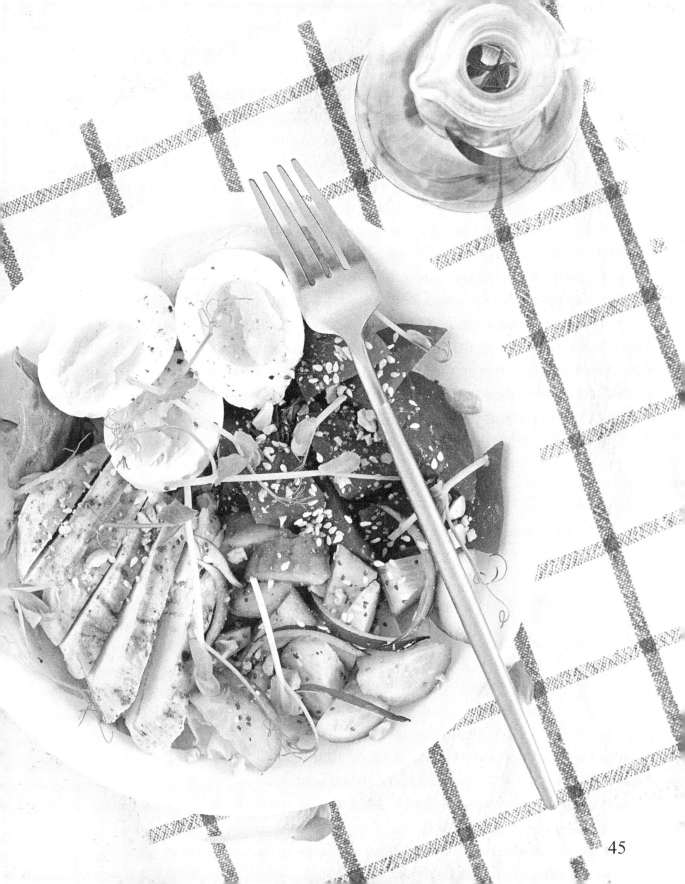

WHAT IS AN INSTANT POT PRESSURE COOKER

So now, let's learn all about the Instant Pot so you can start cooking!

Now that you know how much I love my Instant Pot, you'll want to know just what an electric pressure cooker is. The Instant Pot is an appliance that's a combination of a pressure cooker, slow cooker, rice cooker, and yogurt maker – all in one handy kitchen device.

What parts make up the Instant Cooker? There's an outer pot, which is the base and heat source for the pressure cooker. Inside of this outer pot goes the inner pot, which is made from durable stainless steel. This inner pot is where all the cooking happens.

There's a lid that goes on top of the inner pot, with a silicone ring that seals tightly to keep food, liquids, and pressure securely in the pot.

On top of the lid are the pressure release and the float valve. The pressure release does just that – it releases pressure from inside the Instant Pot. The float valve on the lid pops up when the Instant Pot is pressurized and lowers back down when it's not. It becomes safe to open the lid of the inner pot when the float valve is down.

The Instant Pot has a condensation collector on the side of the base unit that can be removed. Its purpose is to collect condensation, usually when the Instant Pot is being used as a slow cooker.

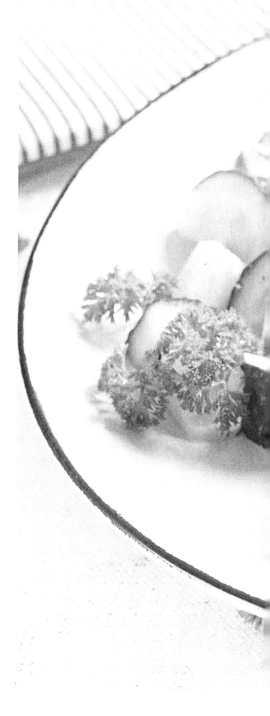

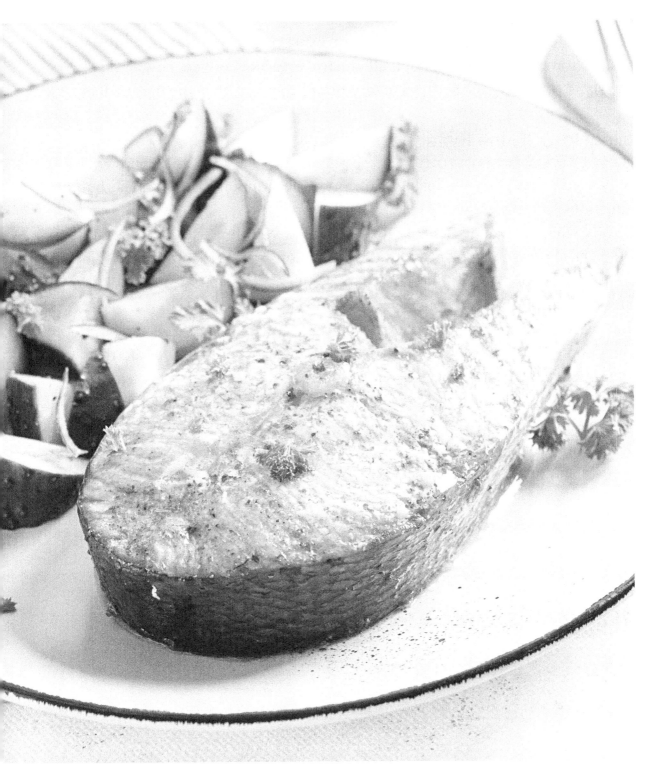

With regard to the Instant Pot's model you possess, it may come with some useful accessories – a steaming rack, measuring cup, and a set of spoons.Not a complex appliance at all, right?

Get to know your brand of Instant Pot by taking a few minutes to read the instruction manual. Even though all electric pressure cookers have pretty much the same functions and settings, every brand comes with some unique features.

How to USE the Instant Pot

When you first get your Instant Pot, don't be intimidated by all the buttons, functions, and programs.

That's what my recipe book is for – to guide you through the steps of using an electric pressure cooker with little confusion. Here are some basic things to know about your Instant Pot that can make it easy for you to start cooking.

Just what is pressure cooking?

Let's get some of the technical information out of the way so you can get to the good stuff... the recipes! The Instant Pot uses a cooking method that seals ingredients and liquids inside a sealed pot. It uses heat to create steam, which then builds up the pressure in the pot. This steam is released or trapped in the pot to control the amount of pressure. With the presence of more pressure, the temperatures will also be higher, and the food cooks faster. Sound complex? Your Instant Pot cooks food fast, fast, fast!

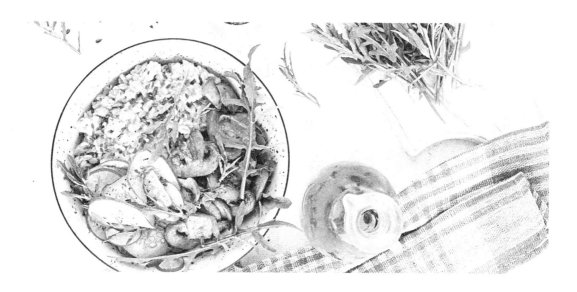

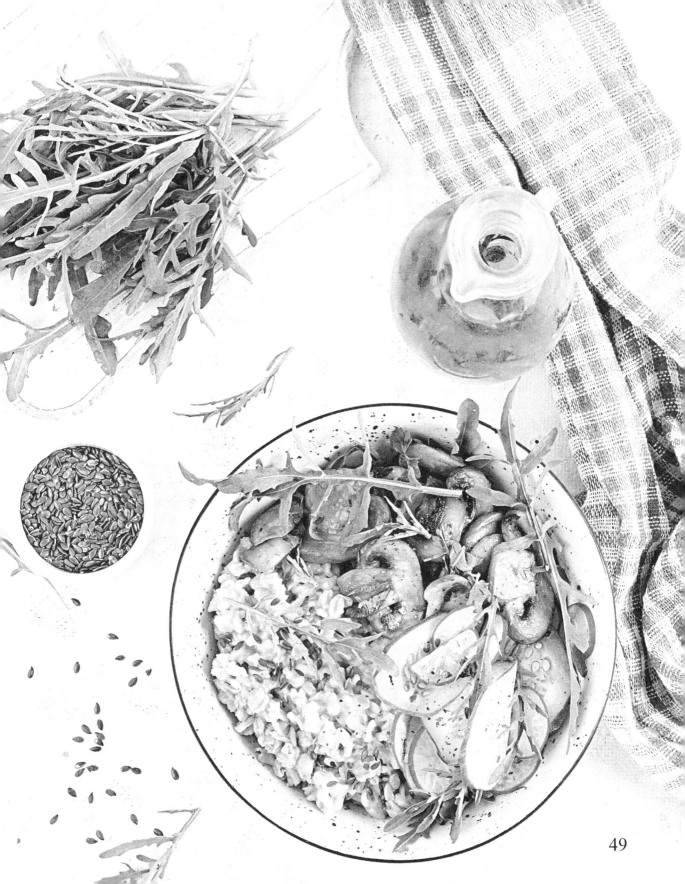

BREAKFAST RECIPES

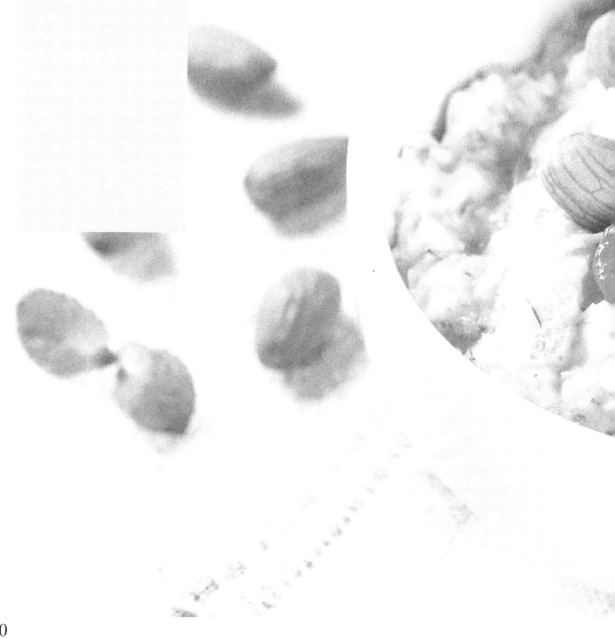

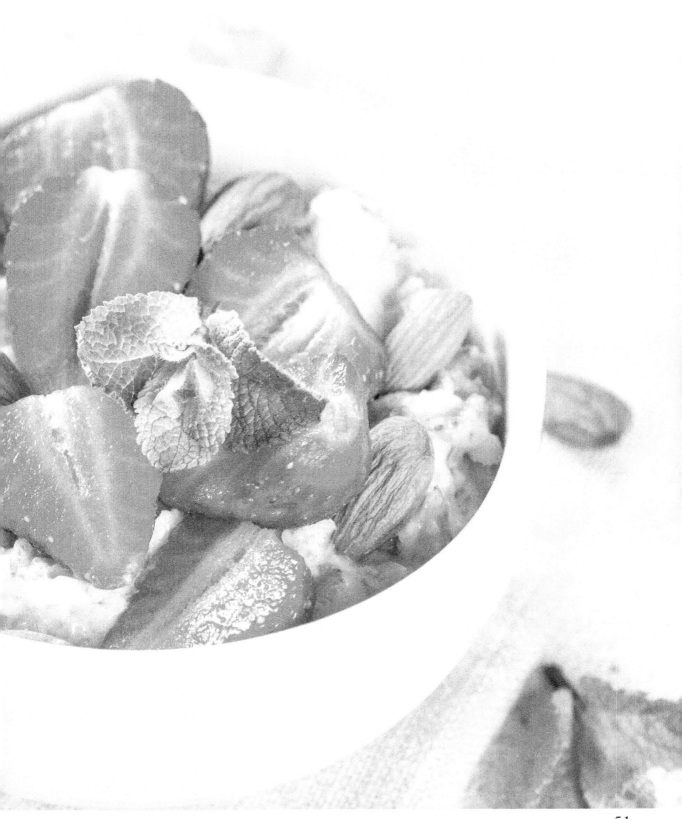

SMOKED PAPRIKA EGGS

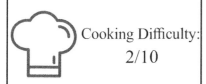 Cooking Difficulty: 2/10

 Cooking Time: 6 minutes

 Servings: 6

INGREDIENTS

- ½ tsp. smoked paprika
- 6 eggs
- ¼ tsp. salt
- pepper
- 1½ c. water

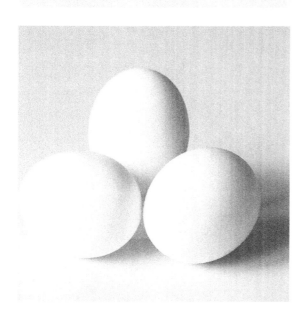

DESCRIPTION

STEP 1
Pour the water into your Instant Pot. Crack the eggs into a baking dish, not breaking the yolks.

STEP 2
Cover the dish with foil and place it on the rack. Close the lid and cook on HIGH for 4 minutes.

STEP 3
Release the pressure quickly and remove the 'loaf' of eggs.

STEP 4
Place on a cutting board and dice the eggs finely. Stir in the spices. Serve and enjoy!

NUTRITIONAL INFORMATION

62 Calories, 4g Fat, 0g Carbs, 2g Protein

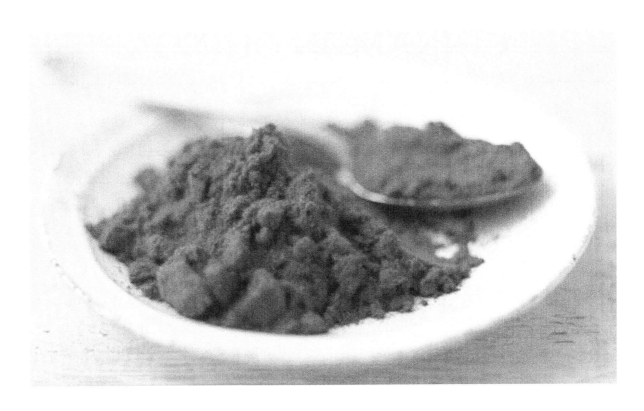

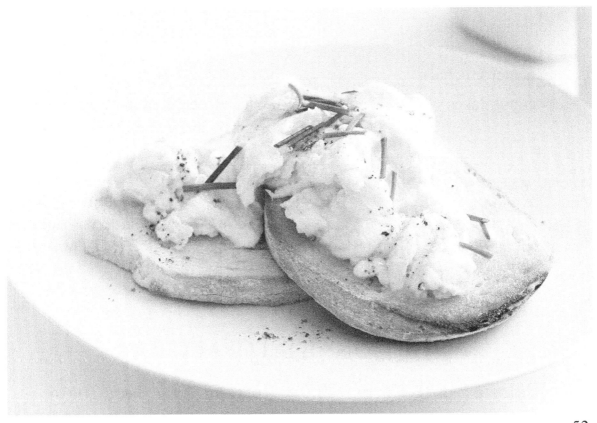

53

CINNAMON QUINOA

 Cooking Difficulty: 2/10

 Cooking Time: 12 minutes

 Servings: 3

INGREDIENTS

- ¾ c. quinoa; soaked in water at least 1 hour
- ½ tsp. ground cinnamon
- 8 oz. almond milk
- ¾ c. water
- 1 tsp. vanilla extract
- 1 pinch salt
  toppings:
- raspberries
- banana (optional)
- coconut flakes

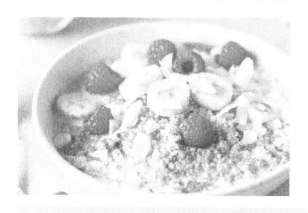

DESCRIPTION

STEP 1
Add all the Ingredients for quinoa to Instant Pot. Secure the lid of instant pot and press *Rice* option.

STEP 2
Adjust the time to 12 minutes and cook at low pressure,

STEP 3
When it beeps, release the pressure naturally and remove the lid.

STEP 4
Stir the prepared quinoa well and serve in a bowl. Add fresh fruits and coconut flakes on top. Add more milk if needed.

NUTRITIONAL INFORMATION

Calories: 370, Carbs: 40.9g, Protein: 7.8g, Fat: 20.6g

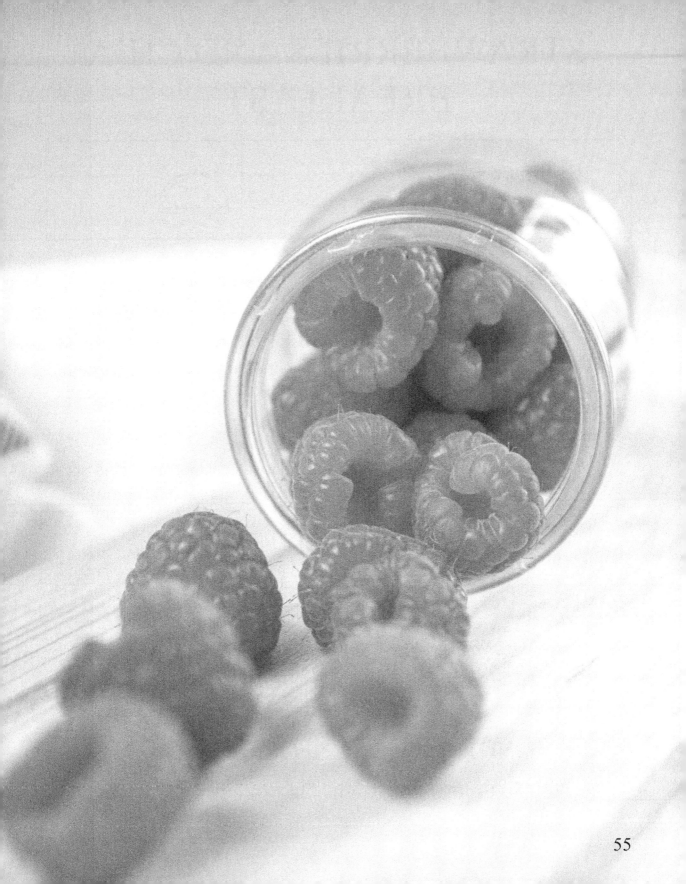

STRAWBERRIES AND CHIA BREAKFAST

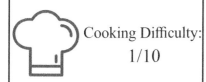 Cooking Difficulty: 1/10

 Cooking Time: 10 minutes

 Servings: 2

INGREDIENTS

- 1 c. brown quinoa
- 4 c. water
- 1 c. oat milk
- 1 c. almonds
- strawberries

DESCRIPTION

STEP 1
In your food processor, mix pepitas with almonds and pulse them well.

STEP 2
In your instant pot, mix chia seeds with water and oat milk and stir.

STEP 3
Add pepitas mix, stir, cover pot and cook on High for 5 minutes.

STEP 4
Add strawberries, toss a bit, divide into 2 bowls and serve for breakfast.

NUTRITIONAL INFORMATION

150 Calories, 4g Carbs, 2g Protein, 1g Fat

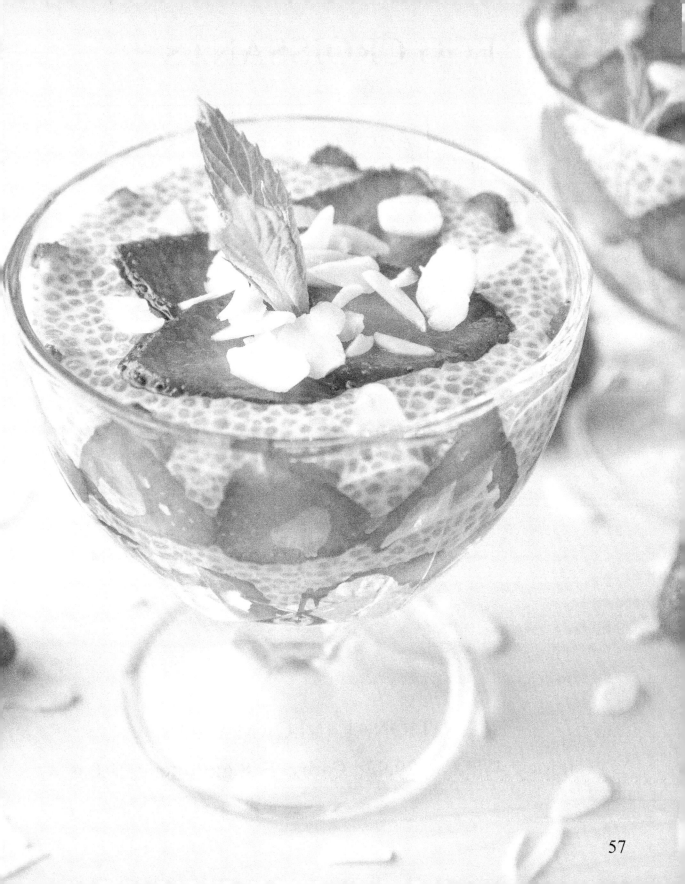

EGG CROISSANTS

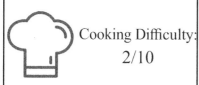 Cooking Difficulty: 2/10	Cooking Time: 10 minutes	Servings: 5

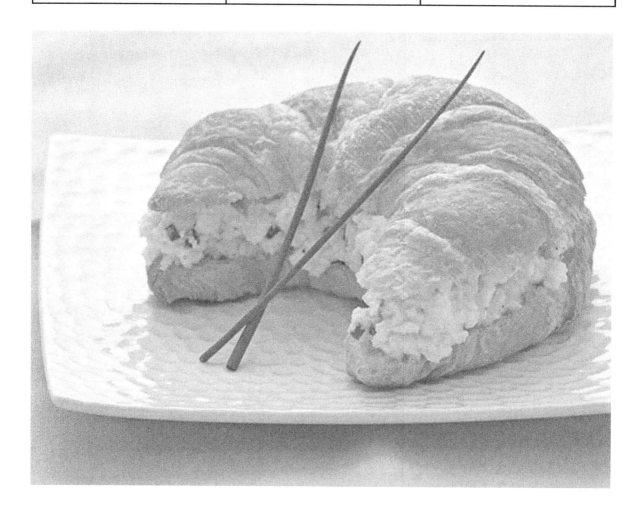

NUTRITIONAL INFORMATION

Calories: 482; Fat: 29.9 g; Carbs: 29.8 g; Protein: 21.0 g

INGREDIENTS

- 5 eggs
- salt
- pepper
- 1 diced green scallion
- 5 croissants

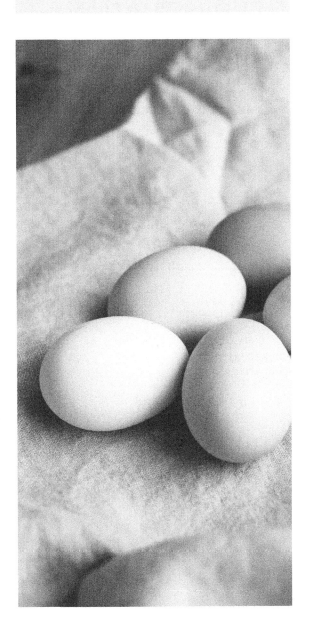

STEP 1
Place a steamer basket inside the Instant Pot and pour in 1½ cups water.

STEP 2
Whip the eggs in a bowl. Add the scallion to the eggs. Mix well.

STEP 3
Divide the mixture into 5 muffin cups. Transfer the filled muffin cups onto the steamer basket.

STEP 4
Shut the lid and cook at high pressure for 8 minutes.

STEP 5
When the cooking is complete, wait a few minutes, and use a quick pressure release.

STEP 6
Lift the muffin cups out of the Instant Pot.

STEP 7
Slice 5 croissants in half and stuff with the muffin cup content.

CHOCOLATE QUINOA SOUP

 Cooking Difficulty: 2/10

 Cooking Time: 22 minutes

 Servings: 2

INGREDIENTS

- 1 c. brown quinoa
- 4 c. water
- 2 tbsps. dutch cocoa powder
- ¼ c. chopped dark chocolate (optional)
- 1 c. vegan milk

DESCRIPTION

STEP 1
Pour brown quinoa, water, cocoa powder and dark chocolate into the Instant Pot. Stir mixture well.

STEP 2
Close the lid. Lock in place and make sure to seal the valve. Press the pressure button and cook for 8 minutes on high.

STEP 3
When the timer beeps, choose the quick pressure release. This would take 1–2 minutes. Remove the lid. Adjust taste if needed.

STEP 4
To serve, ladle equal portions into 2 bowls. Pour vegan milk.

NUTRITIONAL INFORMATION

Calories: 116; Fat: 4.3 g; Carbs: 14.1 g; Protein: 3.1 g

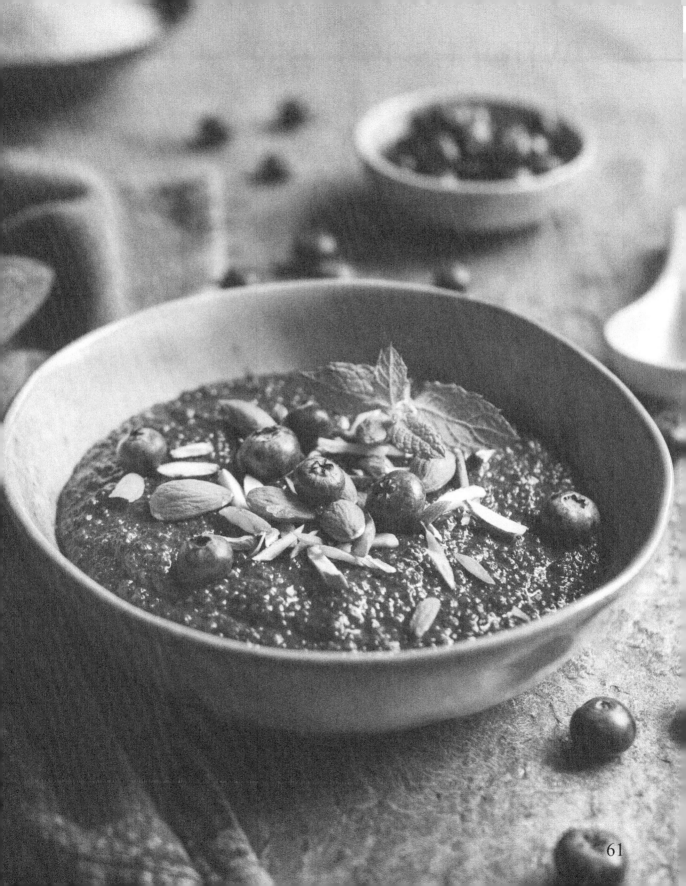

WHOLESOME BREAKFAST EGGS

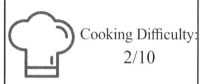 Cooking Difficulty: 2/10	Cooking Time: 7 minutes	Servings: 3

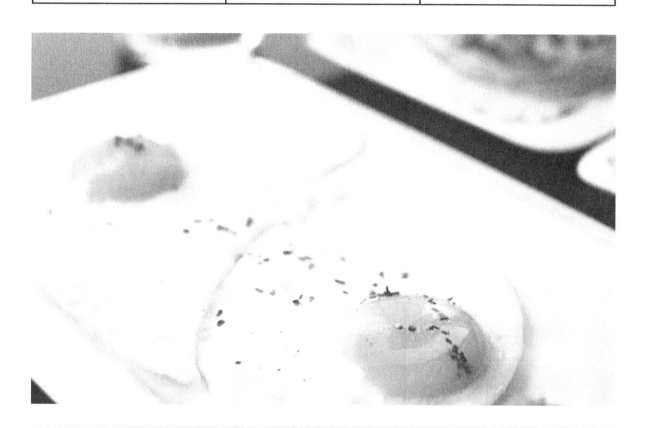

NUTRITIONAL INFORMATION

Calories: 310, Fat: 7g, Carbs: 3g, Protein: 12.5g

INGREDIENTS

- ¼ tsp. cumin, ground
- 6 eggs
- ½ tsp. sea salt
- ¼ tsp. ground cayenne
- 1 tsp. thyme leaves
- 2 chopped garlic cloves
- ½ c. chopped parsley
- ½ c. chopped cilantro
- 2 tbsps. olive oil

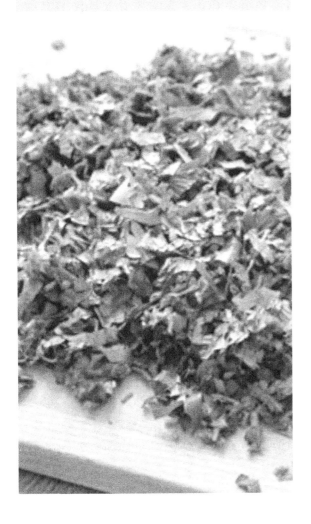

DESCRIPTION

STEP 1
Arrange your Instant Pot over a dry, clean platform. Plug it in a power socket and turn it on.

STEP 2
Now press "Saute" mode from available options. In the cooking area, add the olive oil, and garlic; cook for 2-3 minutes to soften the added ingredients.

STEP 3
Add thyme and cook for a minute. Mix in the parsley and cilantro and cook until it starts to crisp for around 2-3 minutes.

STEP 4
Take the eggs and break into the pan; do not to break the yolks.

STEP 5
Close the lid and lock. Ensure that you have sealed the valve to avoid leakage.

STEP 6
Keep the pot on sauté function and cook for 3 minutes. Open the lid and serve warm!

INSTANT QUINOA

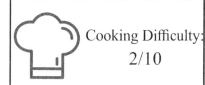 Cooking Difficulty: 2/10

 Cooking Time: 11 minutes

 Servings: 6

INGREDIENTS

- 2 c. quinoa, rinsed
- 2½ c. water
- ½ tsp. vanilla extract
- berries

DESCRIPTION

STEP 1
Add all of the ingredients to the Instant Pot. Stir thoroughly to combine. Cook for 1 minute at high pressure.

STEP 2
When the cooking is complete, do a natural pressure release for 10 minutes. Quick release the remaining pressure.

STEP 3
Open the lid carefully. Serve quinoa with berries.

NUTRITIONAL INFORMATION

383 Calories, 6.2g Fat, 2g Carbs, 5g Protein

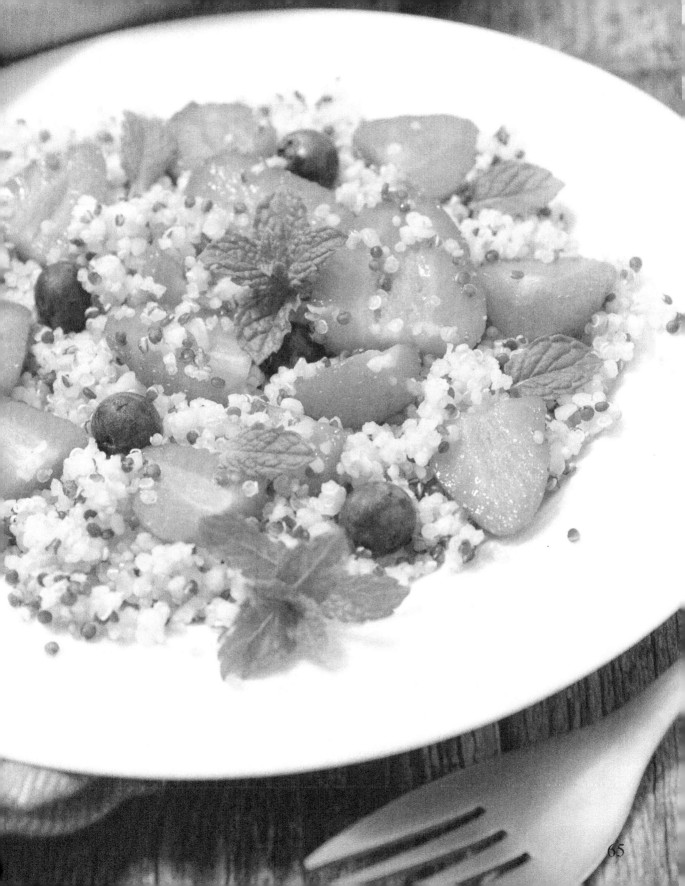

SUNRISE FRITTATAS

Cooking Difficulty: 2/10	Cooking Time: 6 minutes	Servings: 2

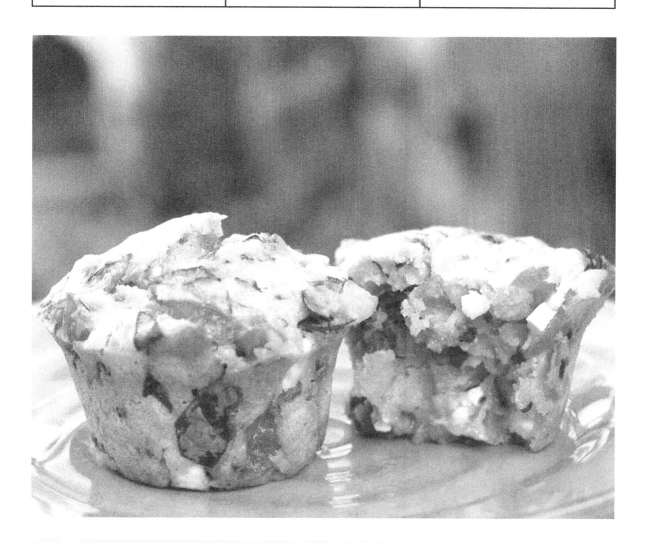

NUTRITIONAL INFORMATION

196 Calories, 4.9g Fat, 4g Carbs, 6g Protein

INGREDIENTS

- 3 eggs
- 2 tbsps. coconut milk
- green onion
- 3 silicon baking molds
- ¼ c. red bell pepper, chopped

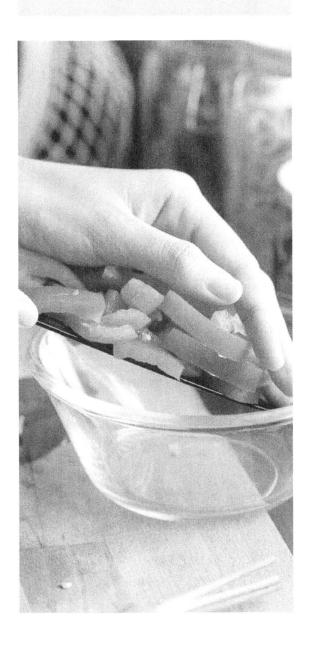

DESCRIPTION

STEP 1
Add 1 cup of water to Instant Pot and place the trivet inside.

STEP 2
Now grease the silicone baking molds with oil and crack an egg into each mold.

STEP 3
Add all the vegetables.

STEP 4
Place the silicone baking molds over the trivet.

STEP 5
Secure the lid of the instant pot and press the *Manual* function key.

STEP 6
Adjust the time to 5 minutes and cook at high pressure

STEP 7
When it beeps; release the pressure naturally and remove the lid. Remove the stuffed molds and serve immediately.

BROCCOLI EGG MORNING

Cooking Difficulty: 2/10	Cooking Time: 9 minutes	Servings: 2

INGREDIENTS

- 3 eggs, whisked
- ½ c. broccoli florets
- ¼ tsp. garlic powder
- 2 tbsps. tomatoes
- 1 minced garlic clove
- ½ chopped yellow onion
- ½ chopped red bell pepper
- 2 tbsps. grated vegan cheese
- 2 tbsps. parsley
- pepper
- salt

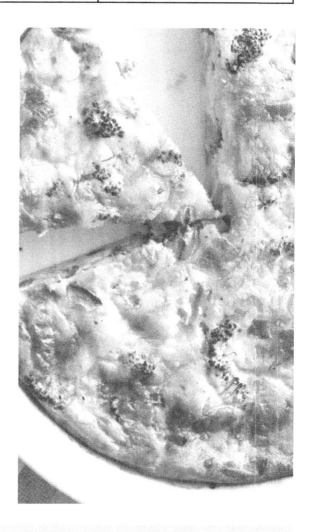

NUTRITIONAL INFORMATION

Calories: 376, Fat: 18g, Carbs: 9g, Protein: 23g

DESCRIPTION

STEP 1

Take your 3-Quart Instant Pot; open the top lid. Plug it and turn it on.

STEP 2

Open the top lid; grease inside cooking surface using a cooking spray.

STEP 3

In a bowl, whisk the eggs. Add the remaining ingredients except for the cheese. Season with Pepper and salt.

STEP 4

In the cooking pot area, add the mixture. Close the top lid and seal its valve.

STEP 5

Press "STEAM" setting. Adjust cooking time to 5 minutes.

STEP 6

Allow the recipe to cook for the set cooking time.

STEP 7

After the set cooking time ends, press "CANCEL" and then press "QPR (Quick Pressure Release)."

STEP 8

Instant Pot will quickly release the pressure.

STEP 9

Open the top lid, add the cooked recipe mix in serving plates. Top with the cheese. Serve and enjoy!

ALMOND AND CHIA BREAKFAST

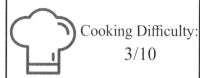 Cooking Difficulty: 3/10

 Cooking Time: 7 minutes

 Servings: 2

INGREDIENTS

- 2 tbsps. chopped almonds
- 1 tbsp. chia seeds
- 2 tbsps. roasted pepitas
- 1/3 c. almod milk
- 1/3 c. water
- a handful blueberries

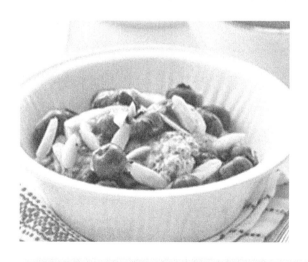

DESCRIPTION

STEP 1
In your food processor, mix pepitas with almonds and pulse them well.

STEP 2
In your instant pot, mix chia seeds with water and almod milk and stir.

STEP 3
Add pepitas mix, stir, cover the pot, and cook on High for 5 minutes.

STEP 4
Add blueberries, toss a bit, divide into 2 bowls and serve for breakfast. Enjoy!

NUTRITIONAL INFORMATION

183 Calories, 6g Fat, 1.8g Carbs, 2g Protein

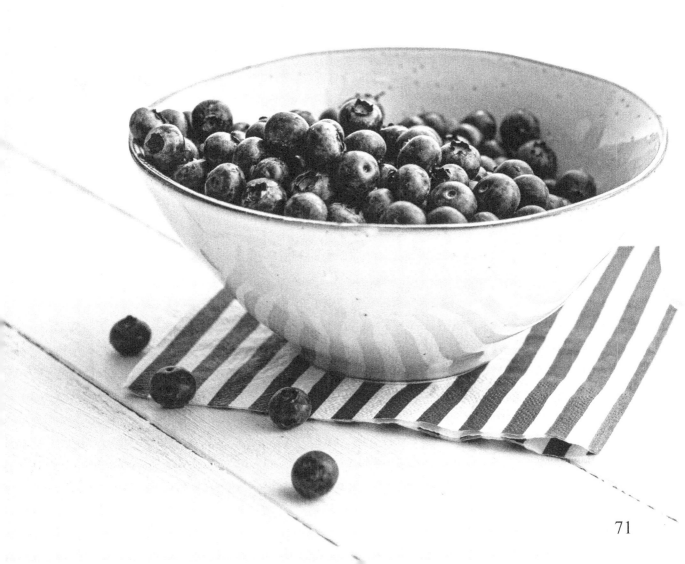

NO-CRUST TOMATO & SPINACH QUICHE

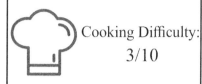 Cooking Difficulty: 3/10	Cooking Time: 32 minutes	Servings: 6

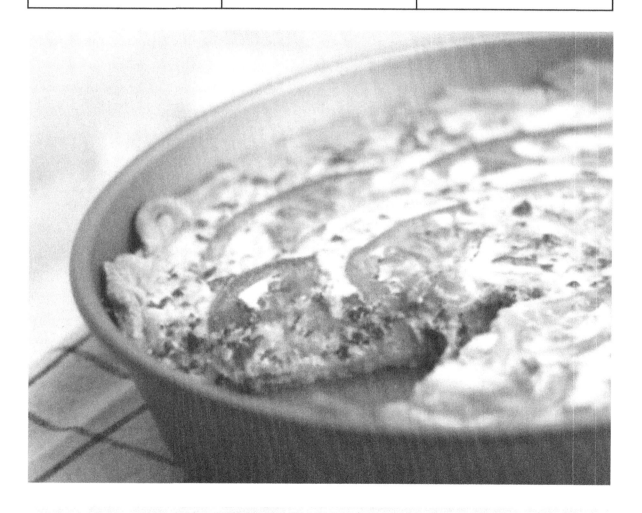

NUTRITIONAL INFORMATION

178 Calories, 3.2g Fat, 3.8g Carbs, 5.3g Protein

INGREDIENTS

- 1 c. diced tomatoes
- 3 c. chopped spinach
- ½ c.coconut milk
- 3 green onions
- 12 eggs
- ½ sliced tomato
- ½ tsp. garlic salt
- ¼ tsp. pepper

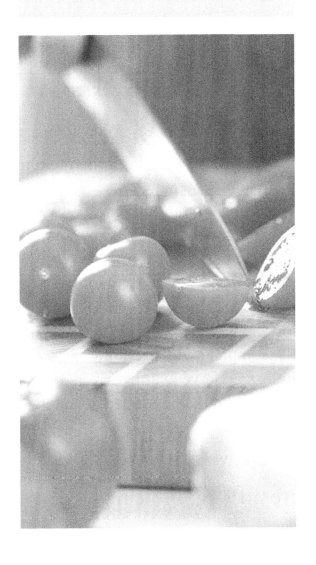

DESCRIPTION

STEP 1
Pour the water into the Instant Pot. Grease a baking dish with cooking spray.

STEP 2
Combine the diced tomatoes, green onions, and spinach in it.

STEP 3
Beat the eggs along with the milk, salt, and pepper.

STEP 4
Pour this mixture over the spinach and tomatoes.

STEP 5
Sprinkle top with tomato slices.

STEP 6
Place the baking dish on the rack and close the lid.

STEP 7
Cook on HIGH for 20 minutes.

STEP 8
Wait 10 minutes before releasing the pressure quickly. Serve and enjoy!

COCONUT OATS

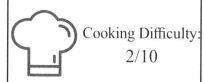 Cooking Difficulty: 2/10

 Cooking Time: 7 minutes

 Servings: 4

INGREDIENTS

- ½ c. coconut flakes, unsweetened
- 1 c. steel cut oats
- 1 c. coconut milk + more for topping
- 2 c. water

DESCRIPTION

STEP 1
Add the coconut flakes to the Instant Pot and select SAUTÉ. Cook for 2–3 minutes, stirring frequently, until lightly brown. Remove half of the coconut to set aside.

STEP 2
Add in oats, toasting until fragrant. Add the coconut milk, reserving some for topping. Stir in the rest of the ingredients. Mix to combine well.

STEP 3
Close the lid and cook at high pressure for 2 minutes. When cooking is complete, do a natural pressure release. Serve warm drizzled with coconut milk and toasted coconut.

NUTRITIONAL INFORMATION

Calories: 218; Fat: 12.3g; Carbs: 19.4g; Protein: 4.4g

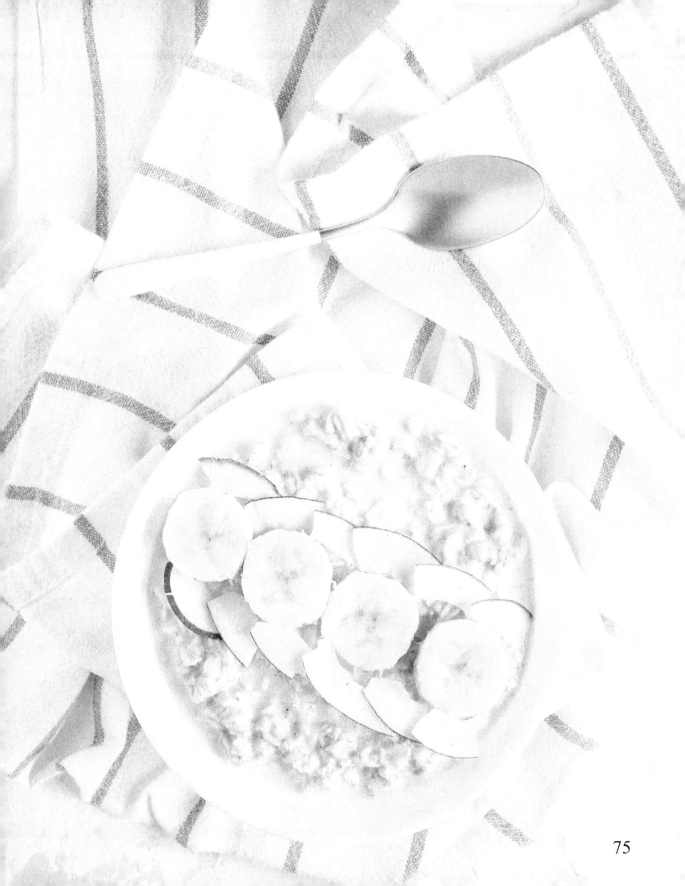

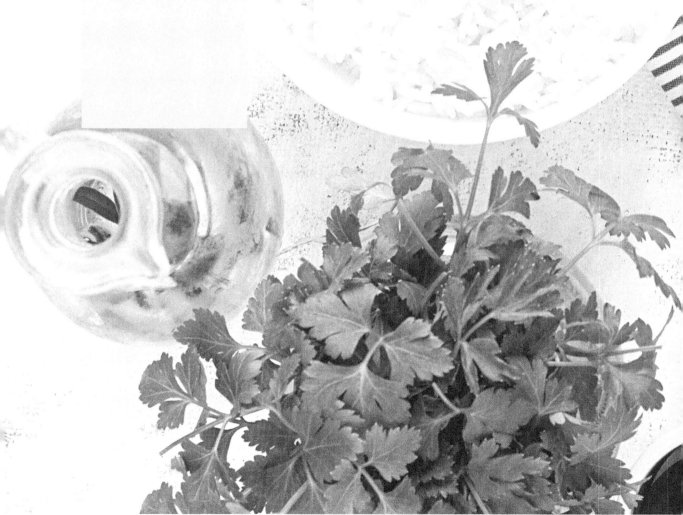

MAIN
DISHES

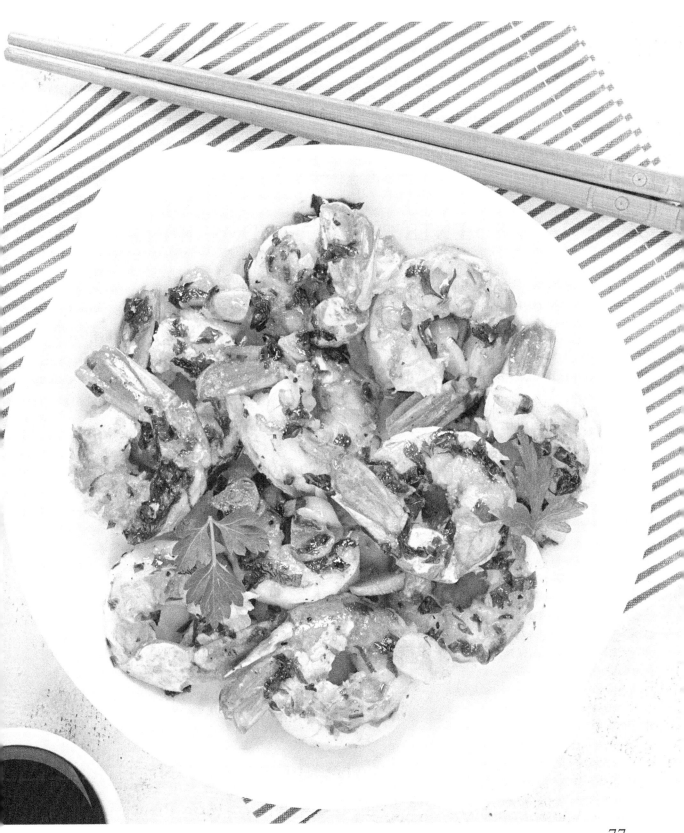

SOCKEYE SALMON

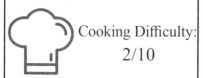 Cooking Difficulty: 2/10	Cooking Time: 6 minutes	Servings: 4

INGREDIENTS

- 4 sockeye salmon fillets
- 1 tsp. dijon mustard
- ¼ tsp. minced garlic
- 1 tbsp. lemon juice
- ¼ tsp. onion powder
- ¼ tsp. lemon pepper
- ½ tsp. garlic powder
- ¼ tsp. salt
- 2 tbsps. olive oil
- 1½ c. water

DESCRIPTION

STEP 1
In a bowl, combine the mustard, garlic, lemon juice, onion powder, lemon pepper, garlic powder, salt, and olive oil. Brush the spice mixture over the salmon fillets.

STEP 2
Pour the water into the Instant Pot. Lower the trivet.

STEP 3
Place the salmon fillets on the rack and close the lid.

STEP 4
Set the Instant Pot to MANUAL and cook at low pressure for 7 minutes. Release the pressure quickly. Serve and enjoy!

NUTRITIONAL INFORMATION

353 Calories, 25g Fat, 0.6g Carbs, 10.6g Protein

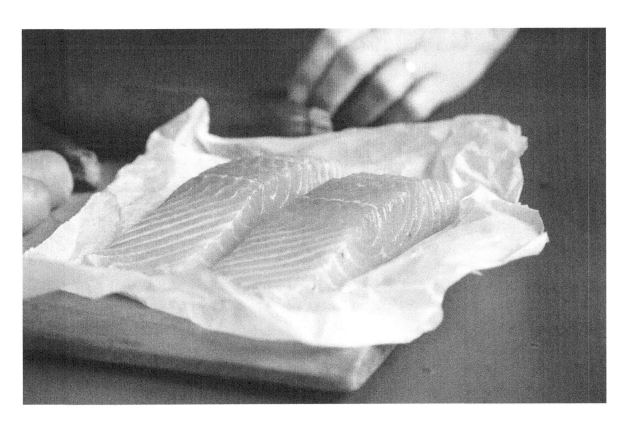

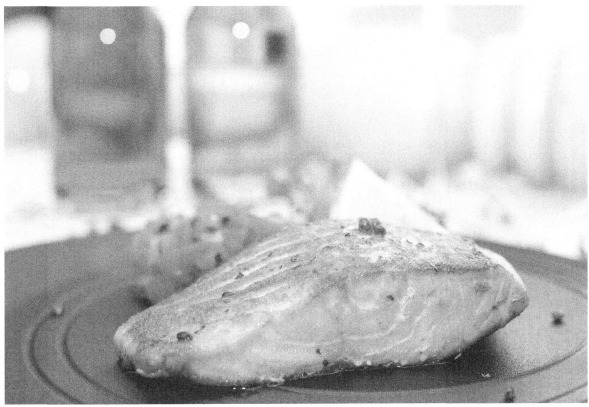

SHRIMP ZOODLES

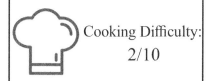 Cooking Difficulty: 2/10	Cooking Time: 10 minutes	Servings: 4

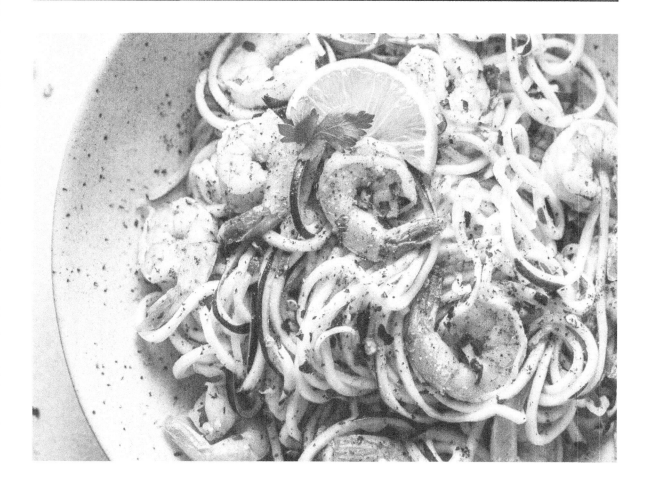

NUTRITIONAL INFORMATION

277 Calories, 15.6g Fat, 5.9g Carbs, 7.5g Protein

INGREDIENTS

- 4 c. zoodles
- 1 tbsp. chopped basil
- 1 lb. shrimp
- 1 c. vegetable stock
- 2 minced garlic cloves
- 2 tbsps. olive oil
- ½ lemon
- ½ tsp. paprika

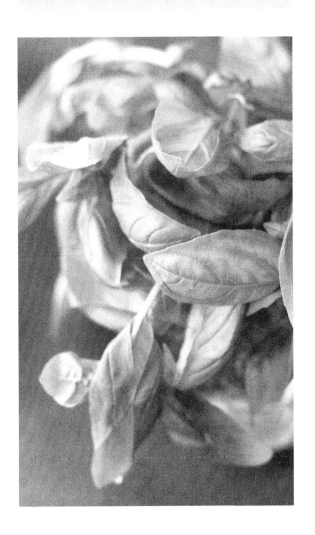

DESCRIPTION

STEP 1
Set your Instant Pot to SAUTÉ and add the olive oil in it.

STEP 2
Add garlic and cook for 1 minute.

STEP 3
Add the lemon juice and shrimp and cook for another minute.

STEP 4
Stir in the remaining ingredients and close the lid.

STEP 5
Set the Instant Pot to MANUAL and cook at low pressure for 5 minutes.

STEP 6
Do a quick pressure release.

STEP 7
Serve and enjoy!

LEMON AND GARLIC PRAWNS

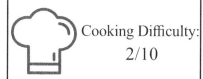 Cooking Difficulty: 2/10	Cooking Time: 7 minutes	Servings: 4

INGREDIENTS

- 2 tbsps. olive oil
- 1 lb. prawns
- 2 tbsps. minced garlic
- 2/3 c. fish stock
- 2 tbsps. lemon juice
- 1 tbsp. lemon zest
- salt
- pepper

DESCRIPTION

STEP 1
Add the oil with the oil in your Instant Pot on SAUTÉ.

STEP 2
Stir in the remaining ingredients.

STEP 3
Close the lid and select the MANUAL option on the Instant Pot. Cook the prawns at low pressure for 5 minutes.

STEP 4
Do a quick pressure release and serve.

NUTRITIONAL INFORMATION

36 Calories, 12.2g Fat, 3.4g Carbs, 7.1g Protein

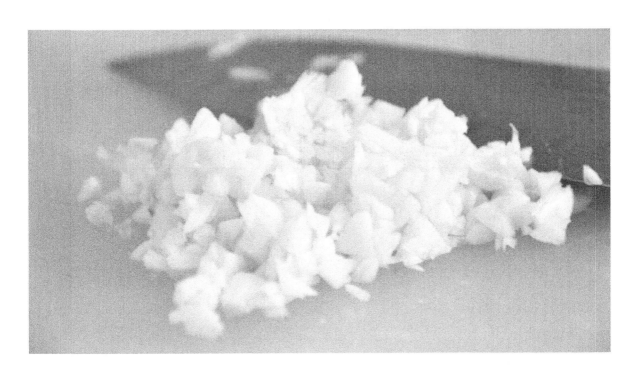

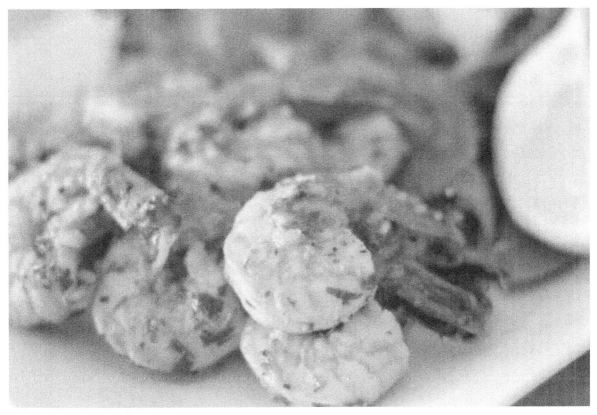

SWEET CORN MIX

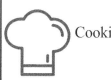 Cooking Difficulty: 2/10

 Cooking Time: 47 minutes

 Servings: 6

INGREDIENTS

- 1 c. sweet corn
- ½ chili pepper
- 3 c. chicken stock
- 1 tsp. olive oil
- 1 tsp. salt
- 1 c. quinoa
- 2 tbsps. sour cream
- 1 onion
- 1 c. sweet pepper
- 2 garlic cloves
- ¼ c. green peas
- 2 tbsps. canola oil

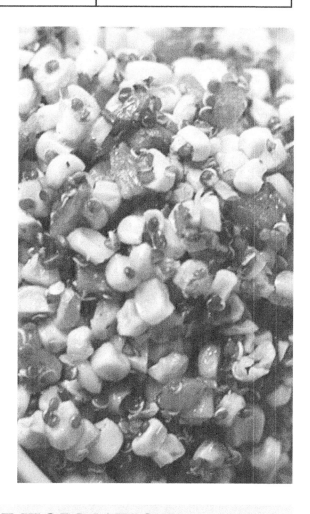

NUTRITIONAL INFORMATION

Calories 389, Fat 24.9g, Carbs 30.21g, Protein 12g

DESCRIPTION

STEP 1
Chop the chili pepper into tiny pieces.

STEP 2
Combine the chili pepper and sweet corn together. Put the quinoa in the instant pot.

STEP 3
Add chicken stock. After this, add olive oil, salt, canola oil, and oregano.

STEP 4
Sprinkle the mixture with the sweet corn mass and stir it carefully with the wooden spatula.

STEP 5
Add sweet pepper.

STEP 6
Peel the onion and dice it.

STEP 7
Add the diced onion and sour cream to the instant pot.

STEP 8
Close the lid and cook the mixture at the sauté mode for 45 minutes

STEP 9
When the sweet corn mix is cooked – put it in the serving bowls. Enjoy!

CHICKEN IN TOMATO SAUCE

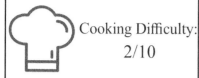 Cooking Difficulty:
2/10

 Cooking Time:
27 minutes

 Servings:
3

INGREDIENTS

- 6 chicken drumsticks
- 1 tbsp. cider vinegar
- 1.5 c. tomatillo sauce
- 1 tsp. olive oil
- 1 tsp. dried oregano
- 1/8 tsp. black pepper
- 1 tsp. salt
- ¼ c. chopped cilantro
- 1 jalapeno, halved and seeded

DESCRIPTION

STEP 1
Season the chicken with salt, vinegar, pepper, oregano and marinate them for 2-hours. Set your instant pot to the sauté mode, add the oil, and heat it.

STEP 2
Saute the chicken until the meat is browned. After frying the chicken, add all the other ingredients (except for the cilantro) and shut the lid to the pot. Set on Manual mode on high, with a cook time of 20-minutes.

STEP 3
When the cooking time is completed, release the pressure using quick-release. Garnish with chopped cilantro just before serving.

NUTRITIONAL INFORMATION
Calories: 302, Fat: 13g, Carbs: 10g, Protein: 32g

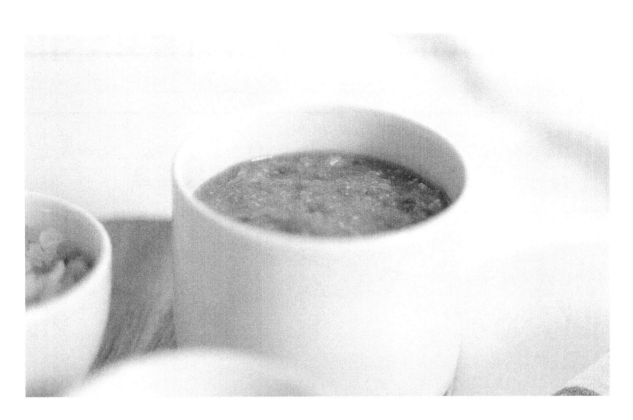

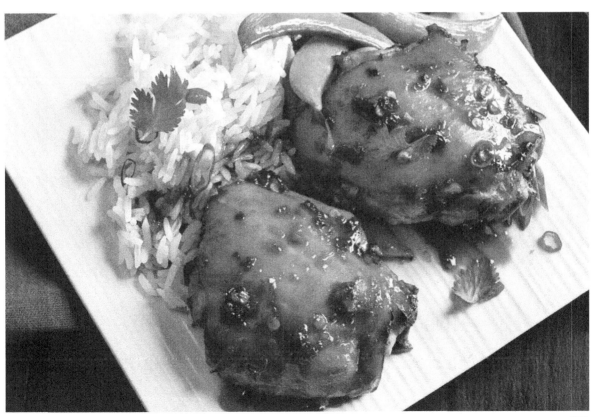

POMODORO SOUP WITH BASIL

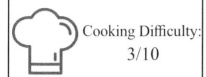 Cooking Difficulty: 3/10	Cooking Time: 20 minutes	Servings: 6

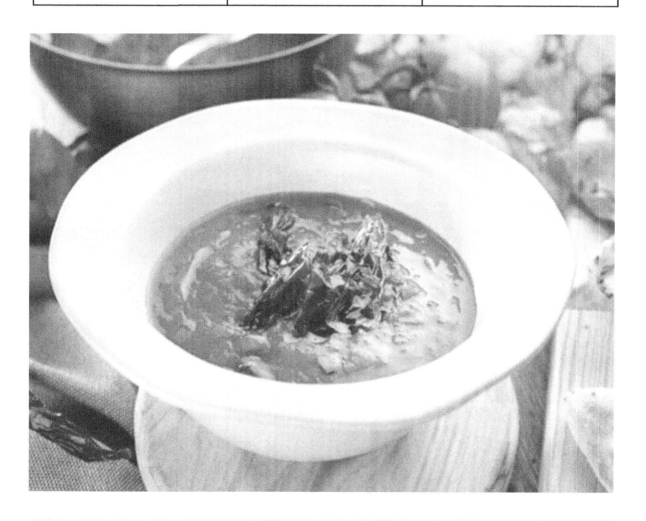

NUTRITIONAL INFORMATION

196 Calories, 13.2g Fat, 4.8g Carbs, 6.4g Protein

INGREDIENTS

- 2 tbsps. olive oil
- ½ diced onion
- 2 tbsps. tomato paste
- 3 c. vegetable broth
- 28 oz. diced tomatoes
- chopped basil
- 1 tsp. balsamic vinegar

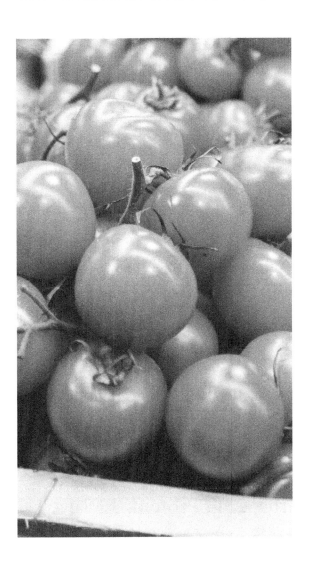

DESCRIPTION

STEP 1
Set your Instant Pot on SAUTÉ and heat the oil in it. Add the onions and sauté for 3–4 minutes.

STEP 2
Stir in the tomato paste and cook for 30–60 seconds.

STEP 3
Pour the broth over and stir in the tomatoes.

STEP 4
Close the lid and cook on SOUP for 10 minutes.

STEP 5
Release the pressure naturally.

STEP 6
Stir in half of the basil and the balsamic vinegar. Use a hand blender to blend the mixture until smooth.

STEP 7
Top with the remaining basil and serve. Enjoy!

QUINOA WITH ACORN SQUASH & SWISS CHARD

Cooking Difficulty: 2/10	Cooking Time: 7 minutes	Servings: 4

INGREDIENTS

- ¾ c. canned acorn squash puree
- ½ tbsp. moroccan seasoning
- 1¾ c. uncooked quinoa, well rinsed
- ½ tsp. sea salt
- 2½ c. water
- ¼ tsp. ground allspice
- 1½ c. swiss chard, trimmed and torn into pieces

DESCRIPTION

STEP 1
Throw all the ingredients into the pot except for the Swiss chard.

STEP 2
Set the pot to Manual mode, on high, with a cook time of 5-minutes.

STEP 3
When the cooking time is completed, release the pressure using quick-release.

STEP 4
Add the Swiss chard and stir, serve right away.

NUTRITIONAL INFORMATION

Calories: 281, Fat: 4.6g, Carbs: 23g, Protein: 12.1g

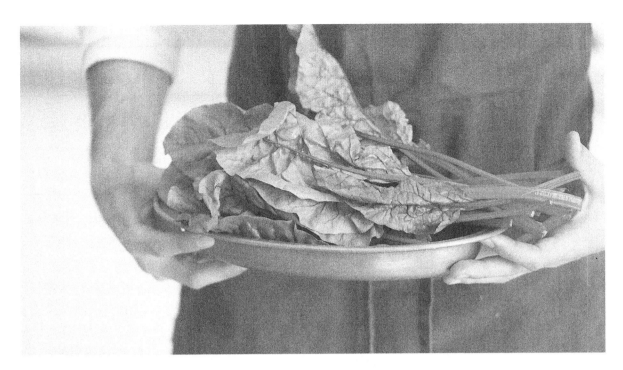

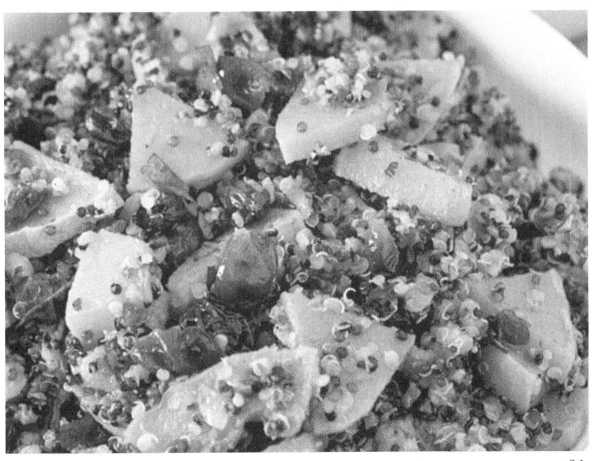

CHICKEN TACOS

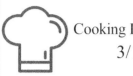 Cooking Difficulty: 3/10	Cooking Time: 32 minutes	Servings: 3

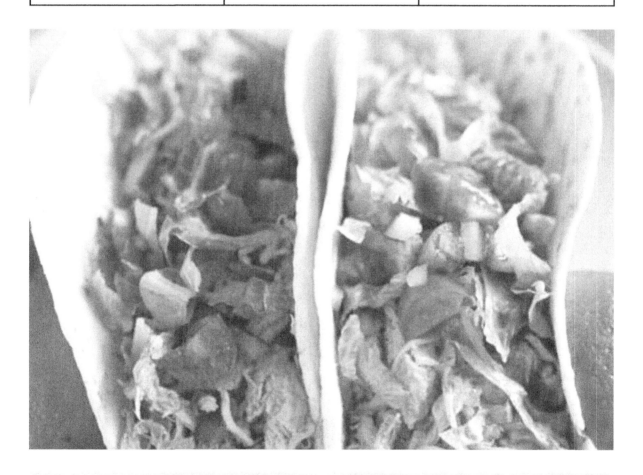

NUTRITIONAL INFORMATION

260 Calories, 2.7g Fats, 30g Carbs, 23.5g Protein

INGREDIENTS

- chicken breast, 6 oz.
- chunky salsa, 1 jar
- taco seasoning, 1 package
- water, ¼ c.
- guacamole
- tortillas

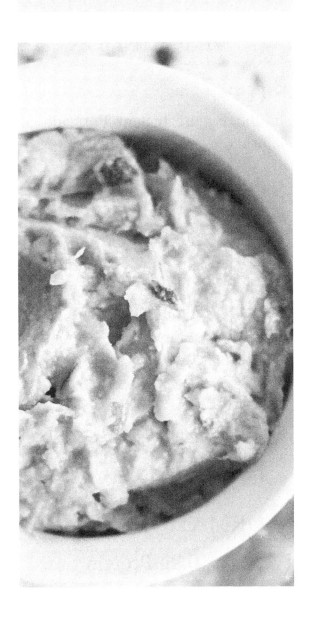

DESCRIPTION

STEP 1
Place the chicken, chunky salsa, Guacamole, taco seasoning, and water into the Instant Pot.

STEP 2
Close the lid and turn the sealing vent to "Sealing."

STEP 3
Select «Poultry» or "Manually High Pressure" and set the cook time for 25 minutes.

STEP 4
Once completed, wait for 5 minutes and then perform a "Quick Pressure Release" by opening the valve to "venting."

STEP 5
Carefully open the lid. Remove the chicken and shred it with a fork.

STEP 6
Return the shredded chicken to your Instant Pot, thoroughly covering it with the sauce. Serve on corn or flour tortillas with your favorite taco toppings!

NICELY FLAVORED SWISS CHARD

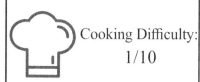 Cooking Difficulty: 1/10	Cooking Time: 5 minutes	Servings: 6

INGREDIENTS

- 2 swiss chard
- 2 tbsps. olive oil
- ¼ tsp. ground cumin
- 1/8 tsp. crushed red pepper flakes
- 1/8 tsp. cayenne pepper
- 1/3 c. water

DESCRIPTION

STEP 1
In the pot of Instant Pot, add all ingredients and stir to combine.

STEP 2
Secure the lid and place the pressure valve to "Seal" position.

STEP 3
Select "Manual" and cook under "High Pressure" for about 3 minutes.

STEP 4
Select the "Cancel" and carefully do a Natural release. Remove the lid and serve.

NUTRITIONAL INFORMATION
50 Calories, 4.8g Fat, 0.31g Carbs, 0.9g Protein

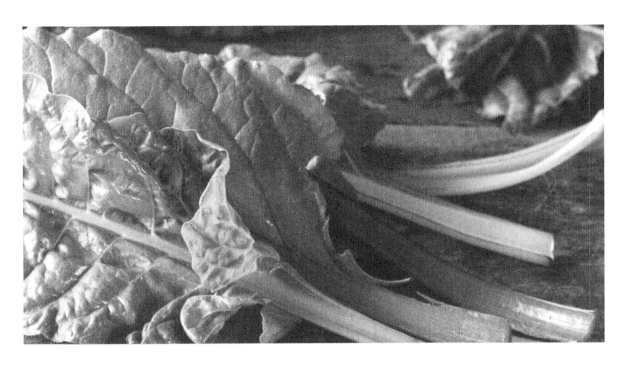

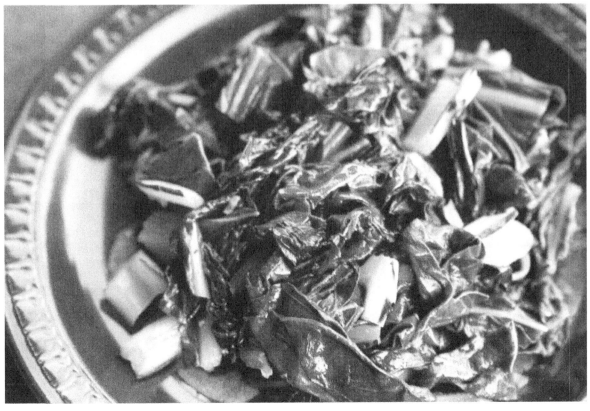

GINGER-SPICED LAMB SHANKS WITH FIGS

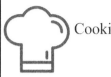 Cooking Difficulty: 3/10	Cooking Time: 98 minutes	Servings: 6

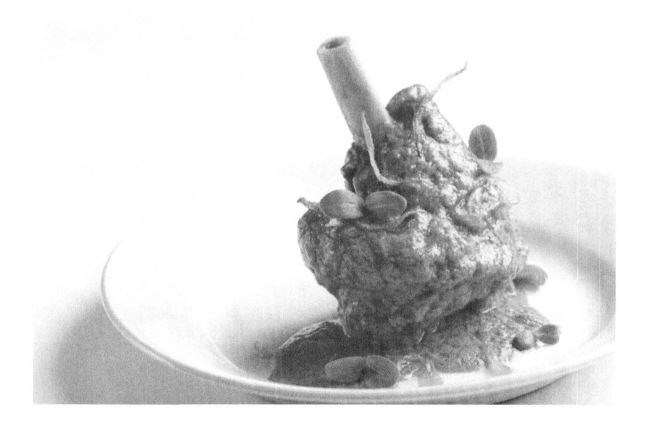

NUTRITIONAL INFORMATION

195 Calories, 14.5g Fat, 5g Carbs, 4.8g Protein

INGREDIENTS

- 4 (12 oz.) lamb shanks
- 1½ c. bone broth
- 2 tsps. fish sauce
- 2 tbsps. apple cider vinegar
- 2 tbsps. ginger, fresh, minced
- 2 tbsps. coconut aminos
- 2 tbsps. coconut oil
- 1 sliced onion
- 3 garlic cloves, minced
- 10 halved and stemmed figs, dried
- salt and pepper

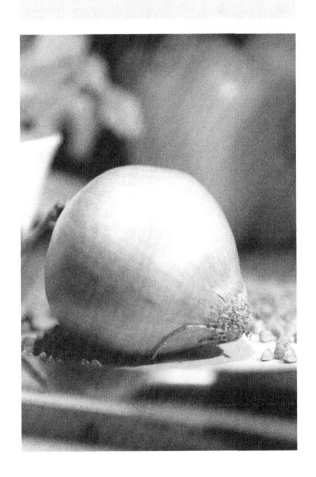

DESCRIPTION

STEP 1
Set your instant pot to the sauté mode, add 1 tablespoon oil, and heat. Add the lamb into the pot and brown on all sides. You might have to do 2 at a time and add more coconut oil.

STEP 2
Place all the lamb shanks on a platter after they are browned. Add the onion and ginger to the pot and stir for 3-minutes.

STEP 3
Add the fish sauce, vinegar, coconut Aminos, and minced garlic. Pour the broth in and add the figs, deglazing any stuck-on meat or onions.

STEP 4
Place the meat back into the pot and close the lid. Set to Manual mode, on high, with a cook time of 60-minutes.

STEP 5
When the cooking time is completed, release the pressure naturally for 30-minutes. Remove shanks from pot, placing them onto serving plates. Add the sauce over the lamb shanks, serve and enjoy!

CHILI ORANGE PRAWNS

Cooking Difficulty: 3/10	Cooking Time: 8 minutes	Servings: 4

INGREDIENTS

- 2 tbsps. olive oil
- 1 lb. prawns
- 2/3 c. fish stock
- 2 tbsps. orange juice
- 1 tbsp. orange zest
- ground chili pepper

STEP 1
Melt the oil in your Instant Pot on SAUTÉ.

STEP 2
Stir in the remaining ingredients.

STEP 3
Close the lid and select the MANUAL option on the Instant Pot.

STEP 4
Cook the prawns at low pressure for 5 minutes.

STEP 5
Do a quick pressure release and serve.

NUTRITIONAL INFORMATION
Calories: 267, Fat: 4g, Carbs: 2g, Protein: 4g

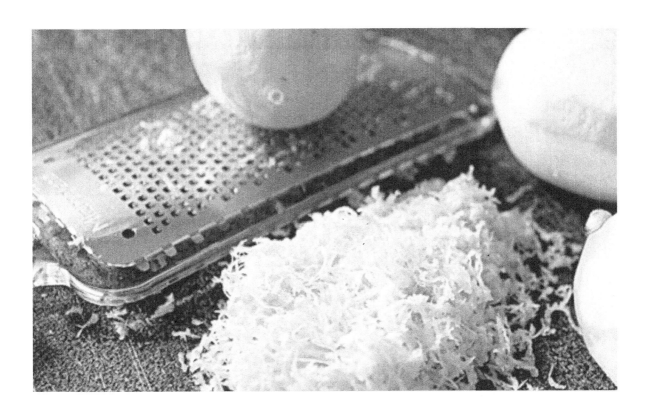

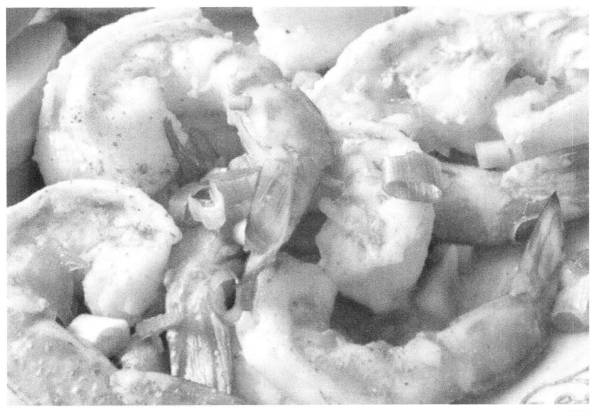

BALSAMIC CHICKEN

 Cooking Difficulty: 3/10

 Cooking Time: 32 minutes

 Servings: 4

INGREDIENTS

- 2 lbs. chicken thigh, skinless and boneless
- salt
- pepper
- ½ tbsp. rosemary
- ½ tbsp. garlic powder
- 1 tbsps. coconut aminos
- 1 tbsp. worcestershire sauce
- 3 tbsps. balsamic vinegar
- 1 c. cranberry sauce
- 1 chopped red onion
- 1 tbsps. cornstarch

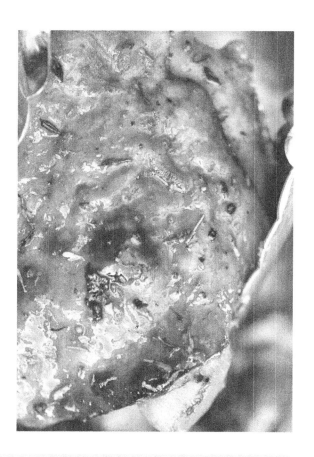

NUTRITIONAL INFORMATION

Calories: 421, Fat: 7g, Carbs: 12g, Protein: 30g

STEP 1

Spray the inside of the instant pot with cooking spray.

STEP 2

Set the pot to the sauté mode. Season chicken thighs with pepper and salt, then transfer to the instant pot.

STEP 3

Brown the thighs for about 5-minutes. Add chopped-up red onion to pot and sauté until caramelized.

STEP 4

Add ¼ cup of water to the pot. In a small mixing bowl, add balsamic vinegar, cranberry sauce, coconut Aminos, rosemary, Worcestershire sauce, and garlic powder, and give it a nice mix.

STEP 5

Close the pot lid, set to Manual mode, on high, for a cook time of 15-minutes.

STEP 6

When the cooking time is completed, release the pressure using the quick-release.

STEP 7

Remove the chicken from the pot.

STEP 8

Add a mixture of 1 tablespoon of water and 1 tablespoon of cornstarch to the sauce in the pot. Sauté for 3-minutes, then pour gravy over the thighs and serve warm.

SPICY HALIBUT IN CUMIN SPICE

Cooking Difficulty: 3/10	Cooking Time: 29 minutes	Servings: 4

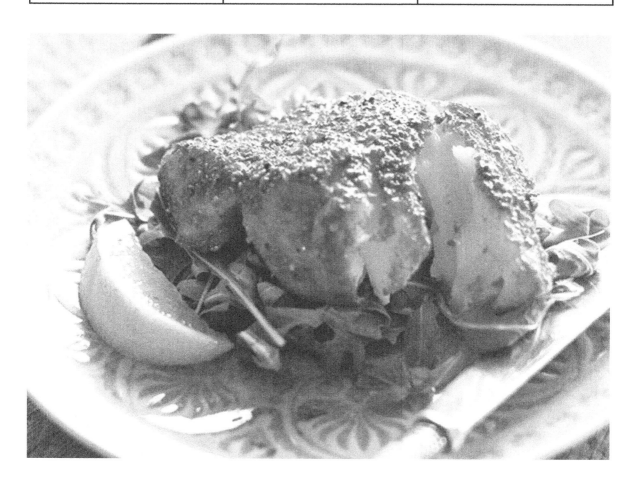

NUTRITIONAL INFORMATION
Calories: 160, Fat: 4g, Carbs: 8g, Protein: 22g

INGREDIENTS

- 4 halibut steaks
- 2 tsp. hot paprika
- 4 garlic cloves
- 1 tsp. dill weed
- 1½ tsp. ground cumin
- 1 tbsp. extra–virgin olive oil
- ½ tsp. black pepper
- 1 orange juice, freshly squeezed

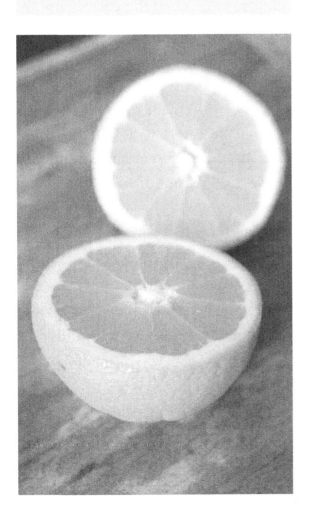

DESCRIPTION

STEP 1
Put together cumin, garlic, orange juice, hot paprika, dill and pepper In a food processor. Process for 1–2 minutes or until all the ingredients are combined well.

STEP 2
Rub processed mixture into the halibut steaks. Allow the mixture to meld and be absorbed by the fish for 25 minutes.

STEP 3
After 25 minutes, layer the fish steaks into the Instant Pot Pressure Cooker. Close the lid carefully. Press the "pressure" button and cook for 5 minutes.

STEP 4
When the timer beeps, choose the quick pressure release. This would take 1–2 minutes. Remove the lid.

STEP 5
Turn off the pressure cooker. Carefully remove the lid. Remove fish and transfer to a platter. Serve with cumin spice mixture on the side.

INSTANT POT LAMB STEW

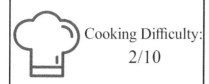 Cooking Difficulty: 2/10	Cooking Time: 27 minutes	Servings: 6

INGREDIENTS

- 2 lbs. lamb stew meat, cubed
- 1 acorn squash
- ¼ tsp. salt
- 6 sliced cloves garlic
- 1 bay leaf
- 2 sprigs rosemary
- 1 large yellow onion
- 3 pieces carrot

DESCRIPTION

STEP 1

Peel the squash and deseed it, cube the squash. Slice the carrots up into circles.

STEP 2

Peel the onion, slice in half and slice the halves into half-moons. Add all the ingredients into an instant pot, close, and secure the pot lid.

STEP 3

Set pot to Manual mode, on high, with a cook time of 25-minutes. When the cooking time is completed, release the pressure naturally for 10-minutes. Serve warm and enjoy!

NUTRITIONAL INFORMATION

Calories: 271, Fat: 20g, Carbs: 5g, Protein: 13g

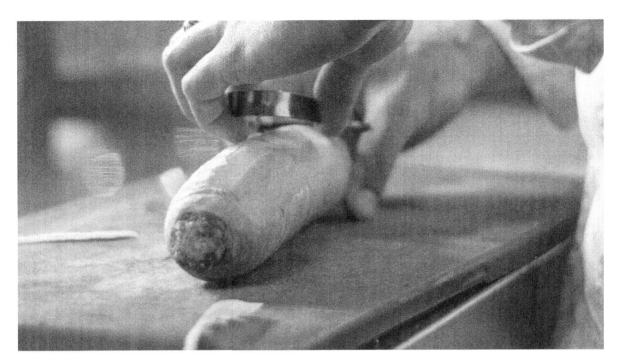

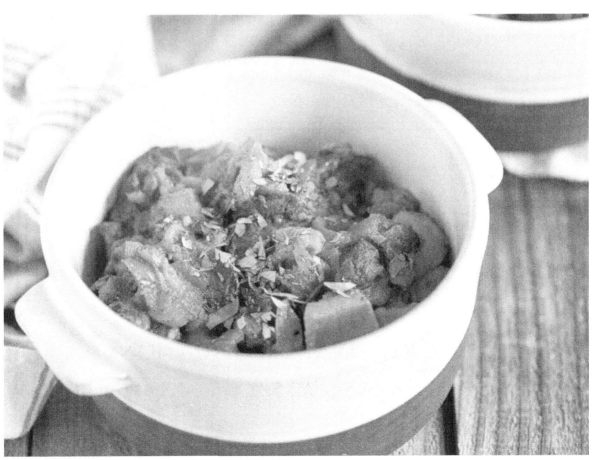

ZESTY BROCCOLI AND CAULIFLOWER BOWL

Cooking Difficulty: 2/10	Cooking Time: 8 minutes	Servings: 4

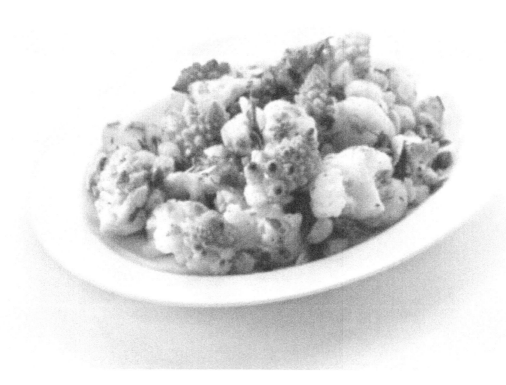

NUTRITIONAL INFORMATION

195 Calories, 14.5g Fat, 5g Carbs, 4.8g Protein

INGREDIENTS

- 1 chopped cauliflower head
- 1 lb. broccoli florets
- 1 tbsp. capers
- 1 grapefruit
- ¼ tsp. pepper
- 4 tbsps. olive oil
- ½ tsp. salt
- 1½ c. water

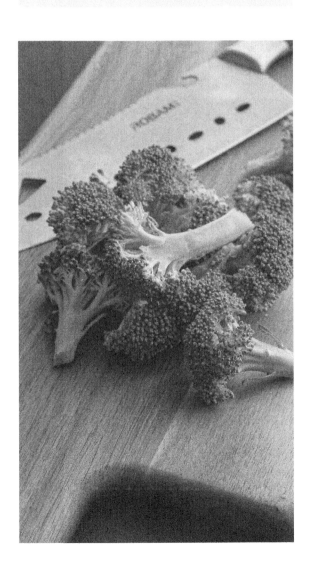

DESCRIPTION

STEP 1

Pour the water into the Instant Pot and lower the steamer basket.

STEP 2

Place the cauliflower and broccoli inside the steamer basket.

STEP 3

Close the lid and Cook on STEAM for 6 minutes.

STEP 4

Meanwhile, place the juice, zest, salt, pepper, capers, and oil in a bowl. Whisk to combine.

STEP 5

Do a quick pressure release and transfer the veggies to a bowl.

STEP 6

Pour the dressing over. Enjoy!

SALMON WITH TOMATO SAUCE

Cooking Difficulty: 3/10	Cooking Time: 12 minutes	Servings: 3

INGREDIENTS

- 6 salmon fillets
- black pepper and sea salt
- 1 tsp. dried parsley
- 1 tsp. dried oregano
- 1 tbsp. coconut oil
- 1.5 c. tomatillo sauce
- 1 chopped and seeded red pepper
- 1 tbsp. apple cider vinegar
- ¼ c. freshly chopped cilantro
- feta

DESCRIPTION

STEP 1
Season the fish fillets with salt, pepper, vinegar, oregano, parsley, and marinate for 2-hours.

STEP 2
Set your instant pot to the sauté mode, add the oil. Add fish fillets and cook for 1-minute on each side.

STEP 3
Set the pot to Manual mode, on high, with a cook time of 10-minutes.

STEP 4
When the cook time is completed, release the pressure using the quick-release. Garnish with fresh chopped cilantro before serving.

NUTRITIONAL INFORMATION
Calories: 284, Fat: 11g, Carbs: 7g, Protein: 22g

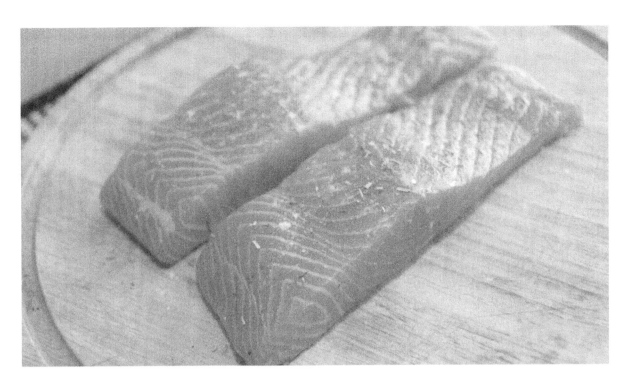

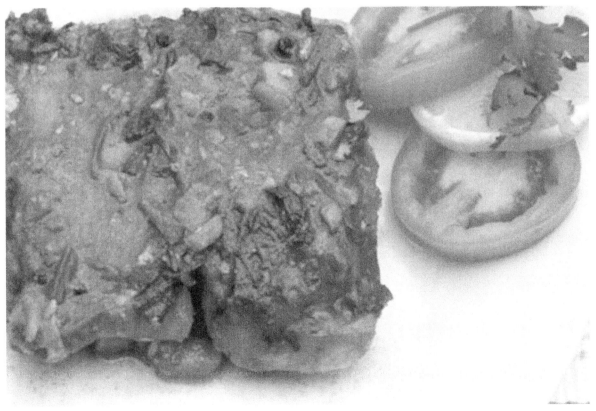

CHICKEN WITH LEMON & COCONUT

Cooking Difficulty: 3/10	Cooking Time: 27 minutes	Servings: 6

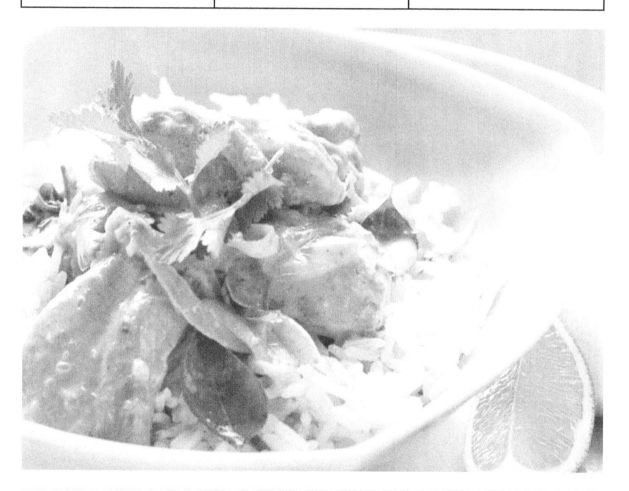

NUTRITIONAL INFORMATION

294 Calories, 18g Fat, 6.1g Carbs, 13.2g Protein

INGREDIENTS

- 1 can coconut milk
- ¼ c. lemon juice
- 1 tsp. lemon zest
- 4 lb. chicken breast
- ½ tsp. salt
- 1 tsp. turmeric

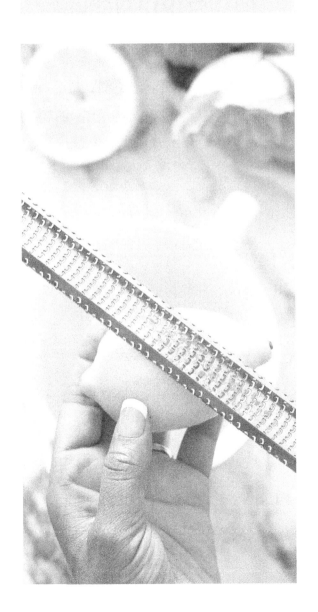

DESCRIPTION

STEP 1
In a bowl, add lemon juice, the liquid portion of coconut milk, lemon zest, and all the spices to make the marinade mixture.

STEP 2
Coat the chicken pieces with the mixture and then set aside.

STEP 3
Pour half the portion of coconut milk into an instant pot, add marinated chicken to the pot.

STEP 4
Pour remaining coconut milk over chicken and close the lid to the pot. Set to the POULTRY setting and cook for 20-minutes.

STEP 5
When the cooking time is completed, release the pressure using the quick-release. Serve the chicken warm as a side dish.

FISH STEW

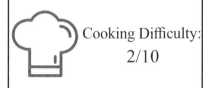 Cooking Difficulty: 2/10

 Cooking Time: 10 minutes

 Servings: 6

INGREDIENTS

- 3 c. fish stock
- 1 diced onion
- 1 c. chopped broccoli
- 2 c. chopped celery stalks
- 1½ c. diced cauliflower
- 1 sliced carrot
- 1 lb. chopped white fish fillets
- 1 c. coconut cream
- 1 bay leaf
- ¼ tsp. pepper
- ½ tsp. salt
- ¼ tsp. garlic powder

DESCRIPTION

STEP 1
Set your Instant Pot to SAUTÉ and add oil in it. Add onion and carrots (if using), and cook for 3 minutes.

STEP 2
Stir in the remaining ingredients.

STEP 3
Close the lid and hit MANUAL. Cook for 4 minutes on HIGH.

STEP 4
Do a natural pressure release. Discard the bay leaf. Serve and enjoy!

NUTRITIONAL INFORMATION

294 Calories, 18g Fat, 6.1g Carbs, 13.2g Protein

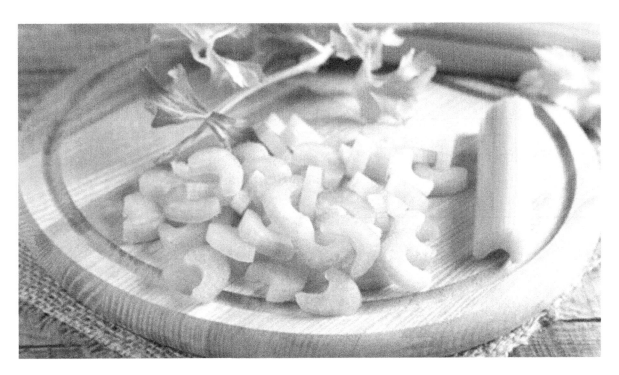

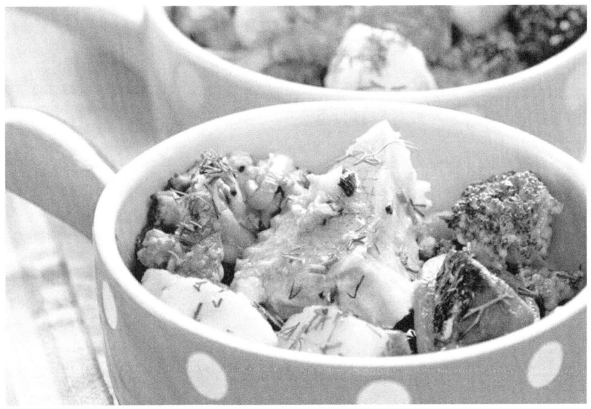

113

DIJON AND LEMON ARTICHOKES

Cooking Difficulty: 3/10	Cooking Time: 33 minutes	Servings: 4

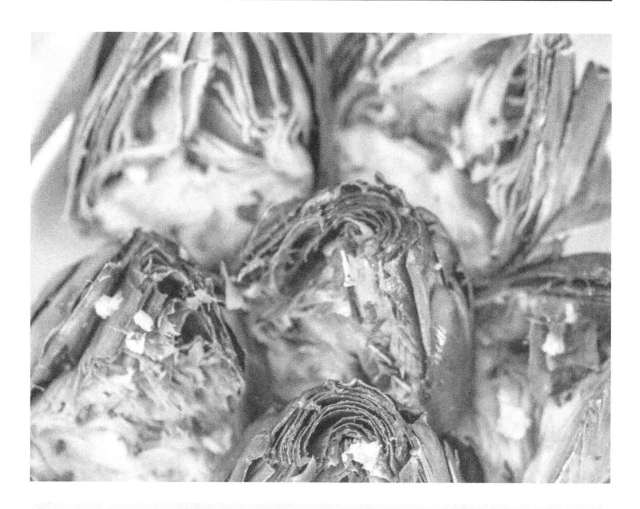

NUTRITIONAL INFORMATION

108 Calories, 7.5g Fat, 2.4g Carbs, 3.1g Protein

INGREDIENTS

- 1½ c. water
- 2 artichokes
- 1 lemon
- ¼ tsp. salt
- ¼ tsp. pepper
- 2 tbsps. dijon mustard
- 2 tbsps. olive oil
- 1 lemon wedge

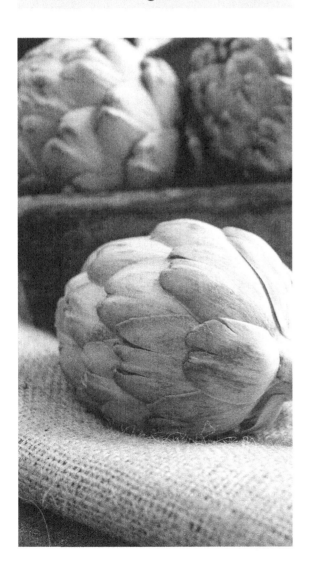

DESCRIPTION

STEP 1
Wash the artichokes well and trim them. Rub them with the lemon wedge.

STEP 2
Pour the water into the Instant Pot and lower the steamer basket.

STEP 3
Place the artichokes in the basket.

STEP 4
Close the lid and cook for 20 minutes on HIGH.

STEP 5
Do a natural pressure release, about 10 minutes. Quickly release the remaining pressure.

STEP 6
In a small bowl, mix together the lemon juice, mustard, olive oil, salt, and pepper.

STEP 7
Serve artichokes with the sauce. Enjoy!

PESTO CHICKEN PASTA

Cooking Difficulty: 3/10	Cooking Time: 12 minutes	Servings: 4

INGREDIENTS

- 4 chicken breasts
- 2 c. gemelli pasta
- 6 oz pesto
- 22 oz. crushed tomatoes
- 1 c. water
- 2 c. baby spinach
- salt
- pepper

DESCRIPTION

STEP 1
Place the chicken, dry pasta, pesto, tomatoes, water, and baby spinach into the Instant Pot, stir to combine. Season with salt and pepper.

STEP 2
Close the lid and turn the sealing vent to "Sealing." Select "Soup/Stew" or "Manually High Pressure" and set the cook time for 10 minutes.

STEP 4
Once completed, perform a "Quick Pressure Release" by opening the valve to "venting."

STEP 5
Serve and enjoy!

NUTRITIONAL INFORMATION

294 Calories, 18g Fat, 6.1g Carbs, 24.2g Protein

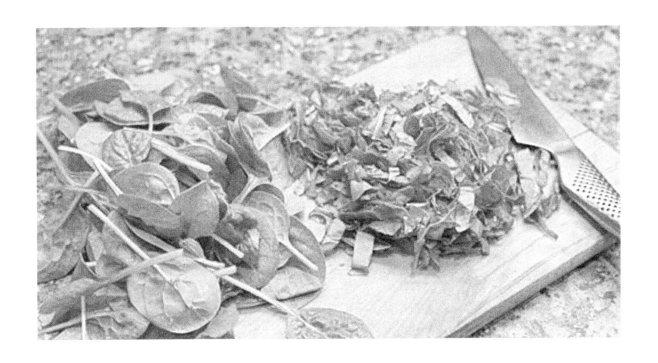

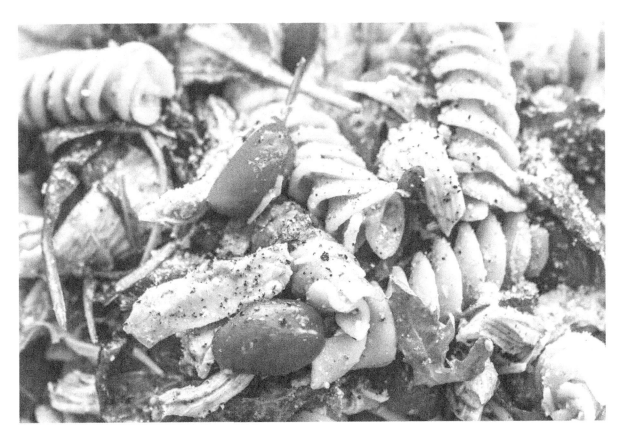

SOUTHERN COLLARD GREENS

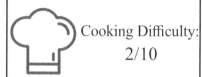 Cooking Difficulty: 2/10	Cooking Time: 13 minutes	Servings: 5

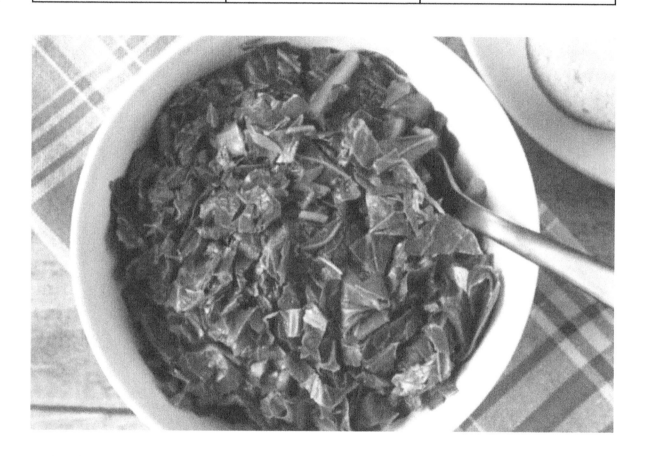

NUTRITIONAL INFORMATION

106 Calories, 6.9g Fat, 2.8g Carbs, 4.3g Protein

INGREDIENTS

- 2 bunches collard greens
- 2 tbsps. olive oil
- 1 yellow onion
- 3 minced garlic cloves
- red pepper flakes
- 1 c. water
- salt

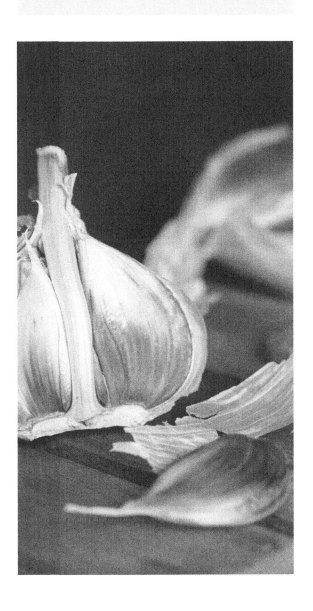

DESCRIPTION

STEP 1
Remove the tough stems of collard greens and then cut them into thin strands.

STEP 2
Place olive oil in the Instant Pot and select "Sauté." Then add the onion and cook for about 4-5 minutes.

STEP 3
Add the garlic and red pepper flakes and cook for about 1 minute.

STEP 4
Select the "Cancel" and stir in collard greens and water.

STEP 5
While the lid is secured, set the pressure valve to the "Seal" position.

STEP 6
Select "Manual" and cook for 3 minutes under "High Pressure."

STEP 7
Select the "Cancel" and carefully do a Quick Release. Remove the lid and stir in salt. Serve hot.

DELICIOUS SALMON FILET

 Cooking Difficulty: 2/10

 Cooking Time: 8 minutes

 Servings: 2

INGREDIENTS

- 2 sockeye salmon fillets
- ¼ tsp. lemon pepper
- ½ tsp. garlic powder
- 1 tsp. dijon mustard
- ¼ tsp. salt
- 1 tbsp. lemon juice
- 2 tbsps. olive oil
- 1½ c. water

DESCRIPTION

STEP 1
In a bowl, combine the mustard, lemon juice, lemon pepper, garlic powder, salt, and olive oil. Brush the spice mixture over the salmon fillets.

STEP 2
Pour the water into the Instant Pot. Lower the trivet.

STEP 3
Place the salmon fillets on the rack and close the lid.

STEP 4
Set the Instant Pot to MANUAL and cook at low pressure for 7 minutes. Release the pressure quickly. Serve and enjoy!

NUTRITIONAL INFORMATION

398 Calories, 28.7g Fats 2.3g Carbs, 30.8g Protein

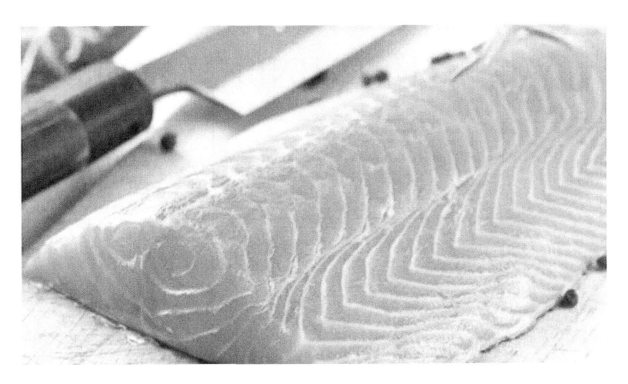

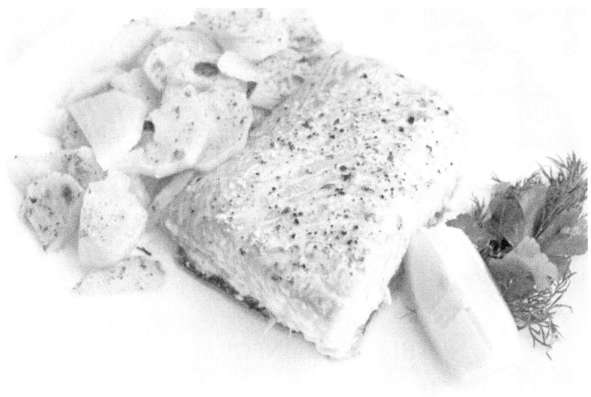

CAULIFLOWER BOLOGNESE WITH ZUCCHINI NOODLES

 Cooking Difficulty: 2/10

 Cooking Time: 8 minutes

 Servings: 2

INGREDIENTS

- 1 medium head cauliflower, broken into florets
- 2 minced cloves garlic
- ½ c. diced onions
- ¾ tsp. dried basil
- red pepper flakes
- 1 tsp. dried oregano flakes
- ¼ c. chicken broth
- 1½ cans (14 oz. each) diced tomatoes
- 3 zucchinis

DESCRIPTION

STEP 1
Add all the ingredients except zucchini to the Instant Pot. Close the lid. Select MANUAL and cook at high pressure for 3 minutes.When the cooking is complete, do a quick pressure release.

STEP 2
Meanwhile, make noodles of the zucchini using a spiralizer using blade A or a julienne peeler.Mash the cauliflower with a potato masher or in a food processor.

STEP 3
Divide the noodles in 4 bowls. Place cauliflower Bolognese over it and serve.

NUTRITIONAL INFORMATION

Calories: 210; Fat: 1.9 g; Carbs: 28.1; Protein: 14.3 g

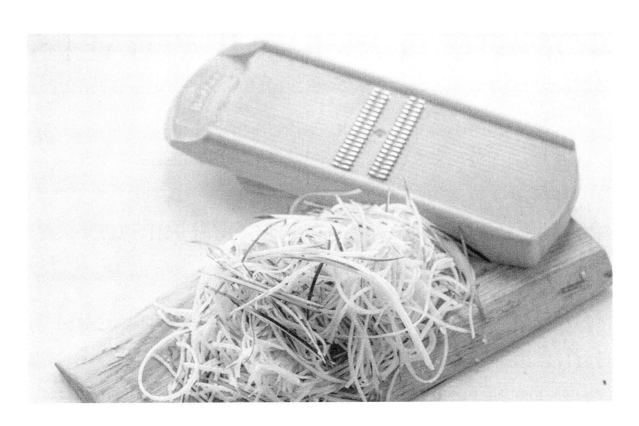

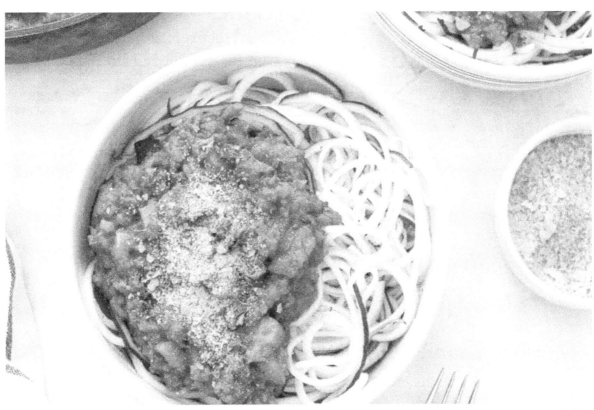

TOMATO TURKEY MEATBALLS

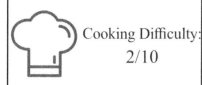 Cooking Difficulty: 2/10

 Cooking Time: 11 minutes

 Servings: 4

INGREDIENTS

- ground turkey, 1 lb.
- diced onion, ¼
- almond flour, 1/3 c.
- garlic powder, ½ tsp.
- chicken stock, ¼ c.
- diced tomatoes, 28 oz.
- olive oil, 1 tbsp.
- basil, ½ tsp.
- pepper, ¼ tsp.

DESCRIPTION

STEP 1
In a bowl, mix the turkey, onion, almond flour until well combined.

STEP 2
Shape the mixture into small meatballs.

STEP 3
Place the remaining ingredients in your Instant Pot and stir to combine.

STEP 4
Place the meatballs inside. Close the lid and set the Instant Pot to MANUAL. Cook on HIGH for 10 minutes.

STEP 5
Release the pressure quickly. Serve and enjoy!

NUTRITIONAL INFORMATION

350 Calories, 20.6g Fats, 6.9g Carbs, 38g Protein

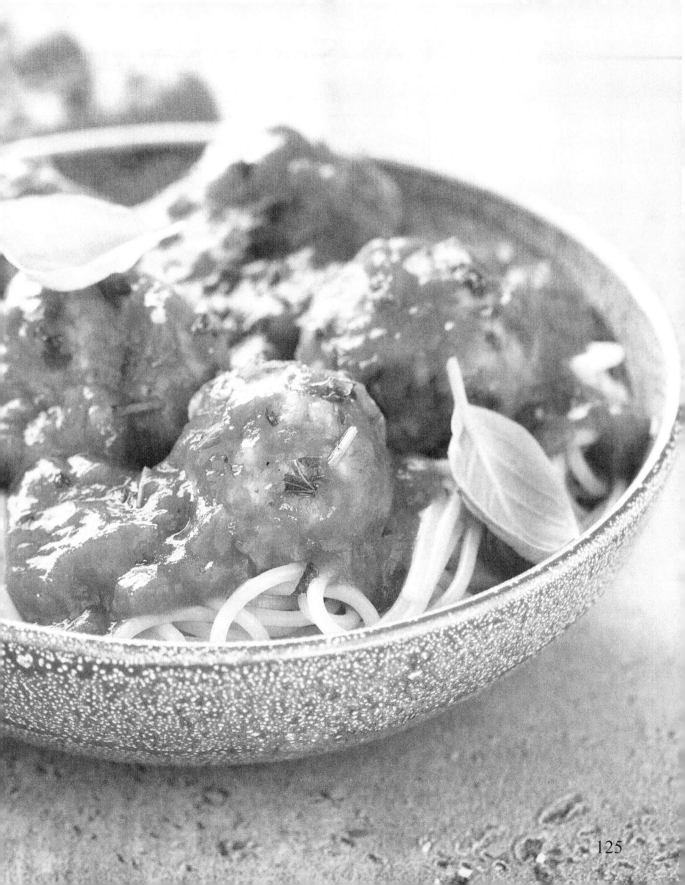

AMERICAN STYLE KALE

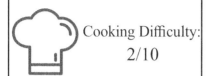 Cooking Difficulty: 2/10	Cooking Time: 10 minutes	Servings: 4

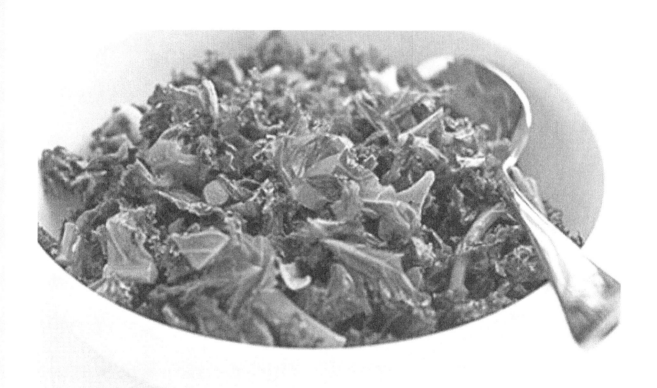

NUTRITIONAL INFORMATION

90 Calories, 12.7g Fat, 3.17g Carbs, 3.6g Protein

INGREDIENTS

- 1 tbsp. olive oil
- 3 garlic cloves
- 1 lb. chopped fresh kale
- ½ c. water
- salt
- black pepper
- 1 tbsp. lemon juice

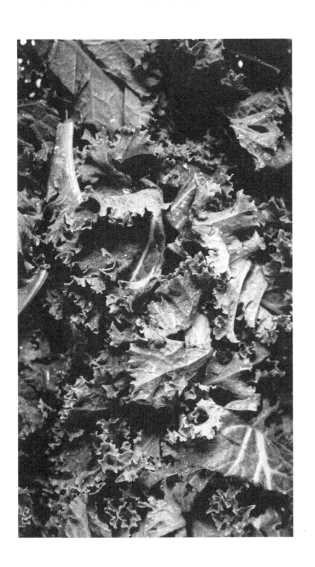

DESCRIPTION

STEP 1
Place the oil in the Instant Pot and select "Sauté." Then add the garlic and cook for about 1 minute.

STEP 2
Add the kale and cook for about 1-2 minutes.

STEP 3
Select the "Cancel" and stir in water, salt, and black pepper.

STEP 4
While the lid is secured, set the pressure valve to the "Seal" position.

STEP 5
Select "Manual" and cook under "High Pressure" for about 5 minutes.

STEP 6
Select the "Cancel" option and do a quick release.

STEP 7
Open the lid and stir in lemon juice. Serve hot.

EGGPLANT ITALIANO

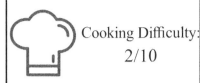 Cooking Difficulty: 2/10

 Cooking Time: 5 minutes

 Servings: 8

INGREDIENTS

- 1½ lbs. eggplant, cubed
- 2 celery stalks, cut into 1-inch pieces
- 2 sliced onions
- 5½ oz. canned tomato sauce
- 2 cans (16 ounce each) diced tomatoes with its juice
- 2 tbsps. olive oil, divided
- 1 c. olives pitted and halved
- 2 tbsps. balsamic vinegar
- 1 tbsps. drained capers
- 2 tsps. dried basil

DESCRIPTION

STEP 1
Add all the ingredients into the Instant Pot. Stir to mix well.

STEP 2
Close the lid. Select MANUAL and cook at high pressure for 4 minutes.

STEP 3
When the cooking is complete, do a quick pressure release.

STEP 4
Garnish with fresh basil and serve over rice or noodles.

NUTRITIONAL INFORMATION
Calories: 127; Fat: 5.8 g; Carbs: 11.6; Protein: 3 g

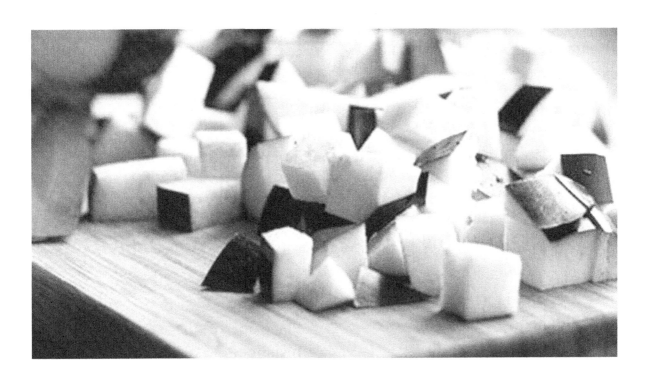

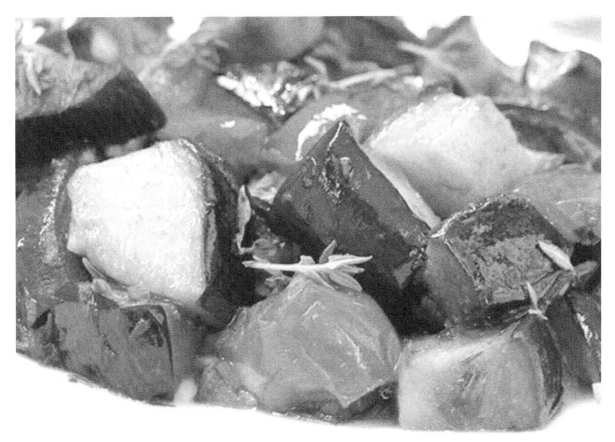

TOMATO WITH TOFU

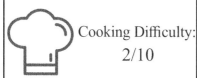 Cooking Difficulty: 2/10

 Cooking Time: 6 minutes

 Servings: 4

INGREDIENTS

- 1 c. diced tomatoes
- 1 cubed block firm tofu
- ½ c. vegetable broth
- 2 tsps. italian seasoning
- 2 tbsps. jarred banana pepper rings
- 1 tbsp. olive oil

DESCRIPTION

STEP 1
Place all of the ingredients in the Instant Pot. Stir to combine the mixture well.

STEP 2
Close the lid and hit MANUAL. Cook for 4 minutes on HIGH.

STEP 3
Do a quick pressure release.

STEP 4
Serve and enjoy!

NUTRITIONAL INFORMATION

68 Calories, 7.4g Fat, 2.3g Carbs, 2.9g Protein

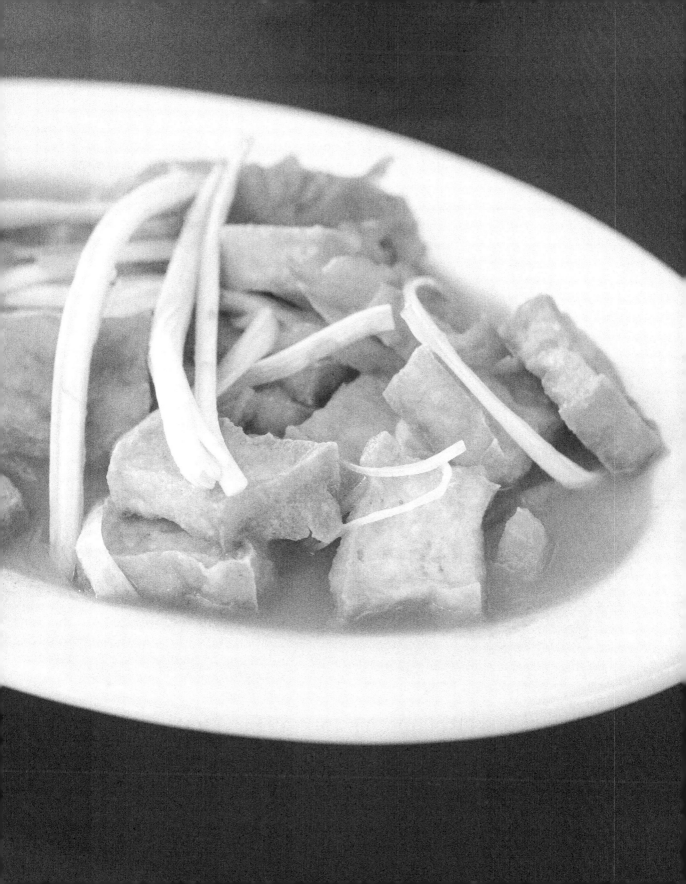

CHERRY TOMATO MACKEREL

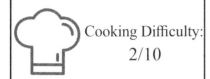 Cooking Difficulty: 2/10	Cooking Time: 10 minutes	Servings: 4

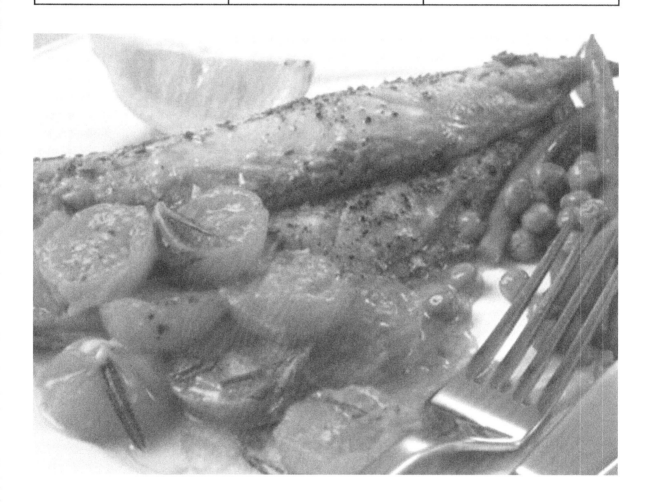

NUTRITIONAL INFORMATION

325 Calories, 24.5g Fat, 2.7g Carbs, 11.9g Protein

INGREDIENTS

- 4 mackerel fillets
- ¼ tsp. onion powder
- ¼ tsp. lemon pepper
- ¼ tsp. garlic powder
- ¼ tsp. salt
- 2 c. cherry tomatoes
- 1½ c. water
- 1 tbsp. black olives

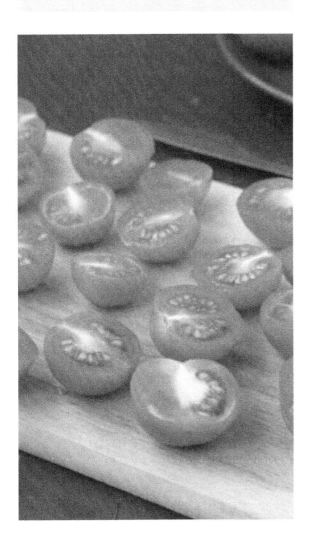

DESCRIPTION

STEP 1
Grease a baking dish that fits inside the Instant Pot with some cooking spray.

STEP 2
Arrange the cherry tomatoes at the bottom of the dish. Top with the mackerel fillets and sprinkle with all of the spices.

STEP 3
Pour water into Instant Pot and lower the trivet.

STEP 4
Place the baking dish on the trivet. Close the lid.

STEP 5
Set the Instant Pot to MANUAL and cook at low pressure for 7 minutes.

STEP 6
Do a quick pressure release.

STEP 7
Serve and enjoy!

MEXICAN CHICKEN SOUP

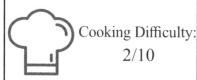 Cooking Difficulty: 2/10	Cooking Time: 13 minutes	Servings: 8

INGREDIENTS

- 2 c. shredded chicken
- 4 tbsps. olive oil
- ½ c. chopped cilantro
- 8 c. chicken broth
- 1/3 c. salsa
- 1 tsp. onion powder
- ½ c. chopped scallions
- 4 oz. chopped green chilies
- ½ tsp. minced habanero
- 1 c. chopped celery root
- 1 tsp. cumin
- 1 tsp. garlic powder
- salt
- pepper

DESCRIPTION

STEP 1
Place everything in the Instant Pot. Give it a good stir to combine.

STEP 2
Close the lid and set Instant Pot to SOUP. Cook for 10 minutes.

STEP 3
When cooking is complete, use a natural pressure release.

STEP 4
Serve and enjoy!

NUTRITIONAL INFORMATION
204 Calories, 14g Fat, 4.2g Carbs, 7.4g Protein

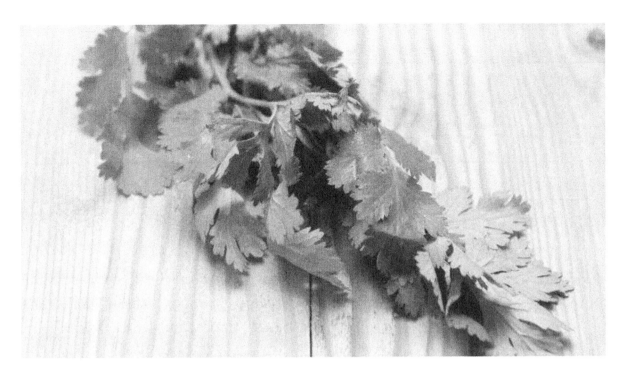

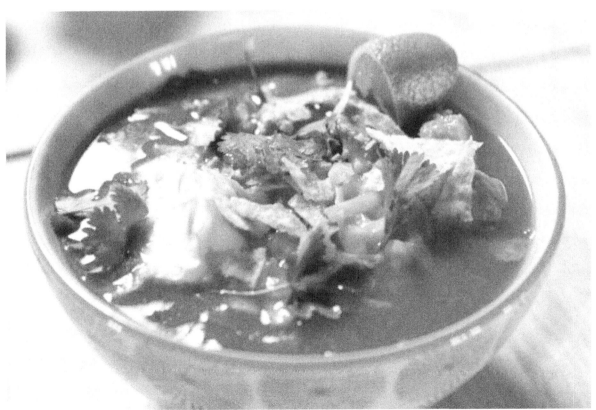

ASIAN BRUSSELS SPROUTS

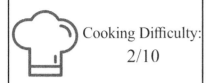 Cooking Difficulty: 2/10

 Cooking Time: 6 minutes

 Servings: 4

INGREDIENTS

- 1 lb. halved brussels sprouts
- 3 tbsps. chicken stock
- salt
- black pepper
- 1 tsp. toasted sesame seeds
- 1 tbsp. chopped green onions
- 1½ tbsps. stevia
- 1 tbsp. coconut aminos
- 2 tbsp. olive oil
- 1 tbsp. keto sriracha sauce

DESCRIPTION

STEP 1
In a bowl, mix oil with coconut aminos, sriracha, stevia, salt, and black pepper, and whisk well.

STEP 2
Put Brussels sprouts in your instant pot, add sriracha mix, stock, green onions, and sesame seeds, stir, cover, and cook on High for 4 minutes. Serve and enjoy!

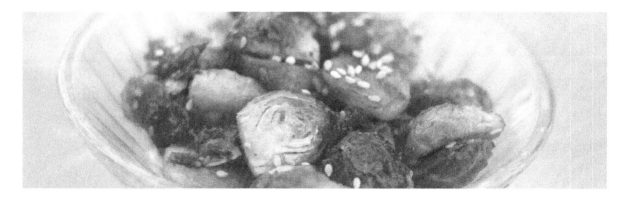

NUTRITIONAL INFORMATION
111 Calories, 4 g Fat, 1g Carbs, 2.2g Protein

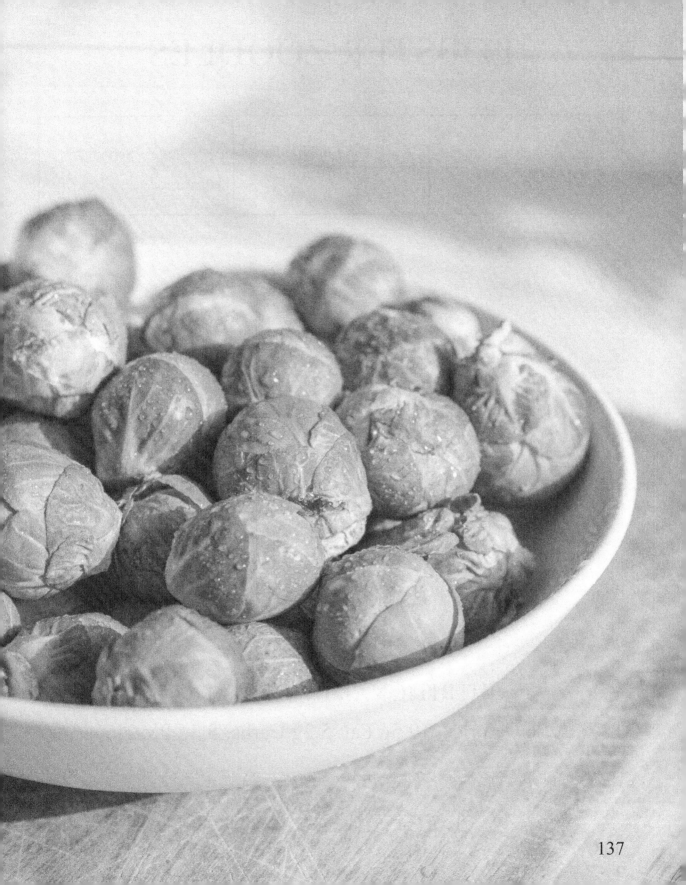

LOBSTER ZOODLES

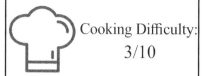 Cooking Difficulty: 3/10	Cooking Time: 10 minutes	Servings: 4

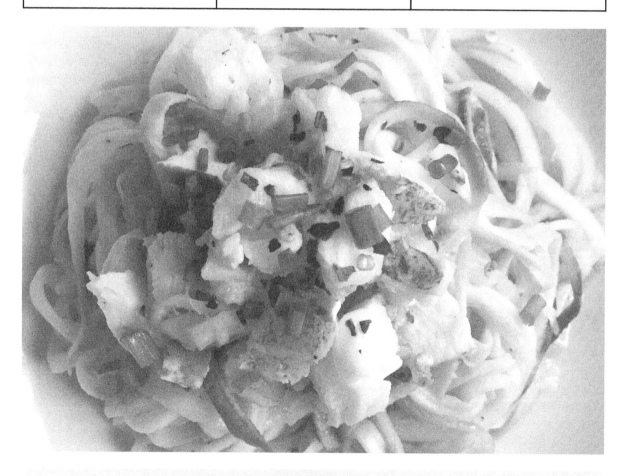

NUTRITIONAL INFORMATION

276 Calories, 19.5g Fat, 5.2g Carbs, 8.3g Protein

INGREDIENTS

- 3 lobster tails
- 1 c. half & half
- 2c. water
- 4 c. zoodles
- 1 tbsp. arrowroot
- 1 tbsp. worcestershire sauce
- ½ tbsp. chopped tarragon

DESCRIPTION

STEP 1
Combine the water and lobster tails in your Instant Pot.

STEP 2
Close the lid and cook for 5 minutes on low pressure.

STEP 3
Do a quick pressure release and transfer the lobster to a plate. Let it cool until easy to handle. Spoon out the meat from the tails and place in a bowl.

STEP 4
Discard the cooking liquid from the pot and combine the Half & Half, arrowroot and Worcestershire sauce in it.

STEP 5
Set the Instant Pot to SAUTÉ and cook the sauce for 2 minutes.

STEP 6
Stir in the lobster and zoodles.

STEP 7
Cook for 3 minutes. Sprinkle with tarragon and serve.

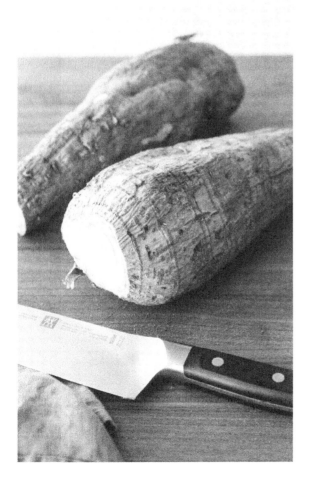

DELICIOUS BROCCOLI SOUP

 Cooking Difficulty: 2/10

 Cooking Time: 30 minutes

 Servings: 2

INGREDIENTS

- 1 chopped broccoli head
- 4 minced garlic cloves
- 3 c. vegetable broth
- 1 c. coconut cream
- 1 tsp. salt
- 1 tsp. black pepper

DESCRIPTION

STEP 1
In your Instant Pot, add broccoli florets, garlic, vegetable stock, coconut cream and salt, black pepper. Stir well.

STEP 2
Close and seal lid. Press the Soup button. Cook for 30 minutes.

STEP 3
Open the lid, blend the mixture with a hand blender, until smooth. Set the pot to SAUTÉ. Let it simmer for 2 minutes. Serve warm.

NUTRITIONAL INFORMATION
Calories: 250; Fat: 25g; Carbs: 5g; Protein: 14g

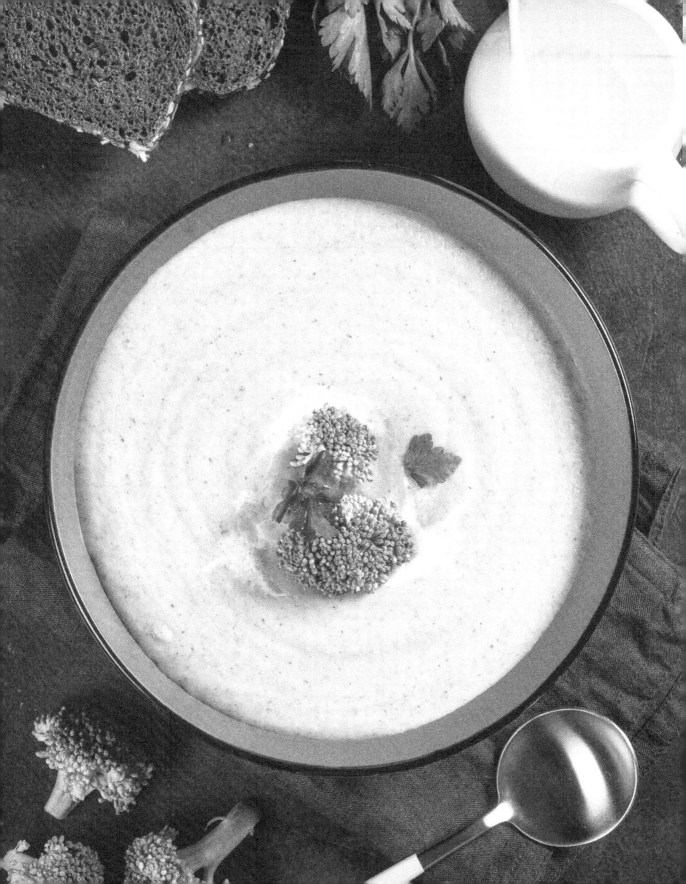

INSTANT CELERIAC AND LEEK SOUP

Cooking Difficulty: 3/10	Cooking Time: 12 minutes	Servings: 6

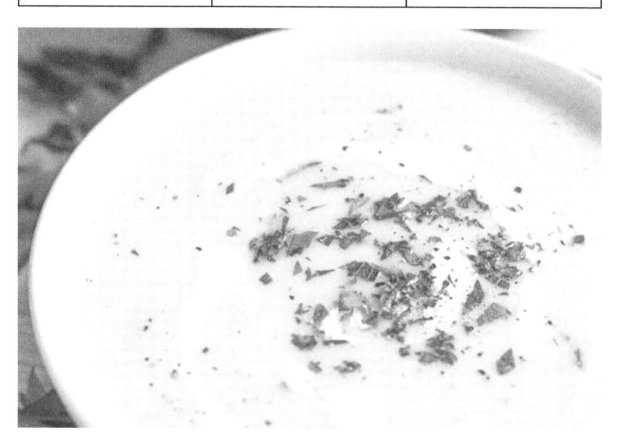

NUTRITIONAL INFORMATION

222.83 Calories, 18.7g Fat, 6.1g Carbs, 1.7g Protein

INGREDIENTS

- 2 tbsps. olive oil
- 2 sliced leeks
- 1 tsp. kosher salt
- 3 crushed cloves garlic
- 3 sprigs thyme, fresh
- 1 tsp. oregano, dry
- 2 leaves bay
- ¾ c. white wine
- 4 c. water
- 4 chopped celeriac root
- 1 c. coconut cream

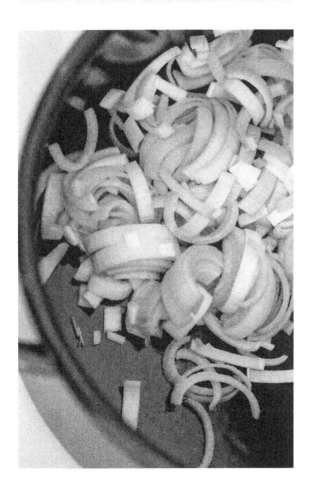

DESCRIPTION

STEP 1
Add olive oil to the Instant Pot. Add leeks and garlic cloves and press saute to soften them.

STEP 2
Kill the heat and set aside.

STEP 3
Add in the bay leaves, celeriac root, thyme, white wine, oregano, and water as you stir.

STEP 4
Select Manual high pressure and wait for 10 minutes.

STEP 5
Open the pot as you select Quick release.

STEP 6
Add the cream puree the soup to obtain a desired rich, creamy consistency.

STEP 7
Serve immediately.

SNACKS & DESSERTS

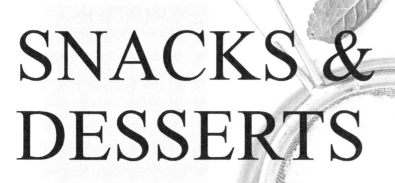

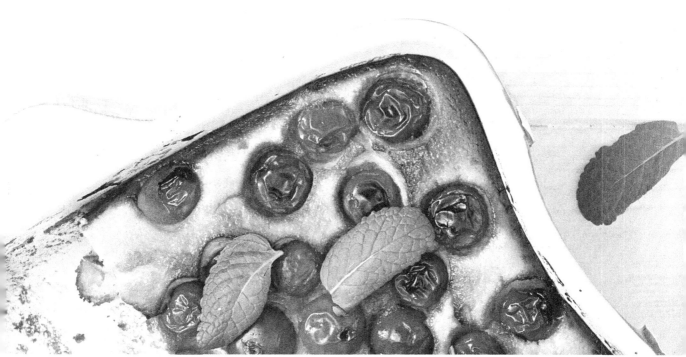

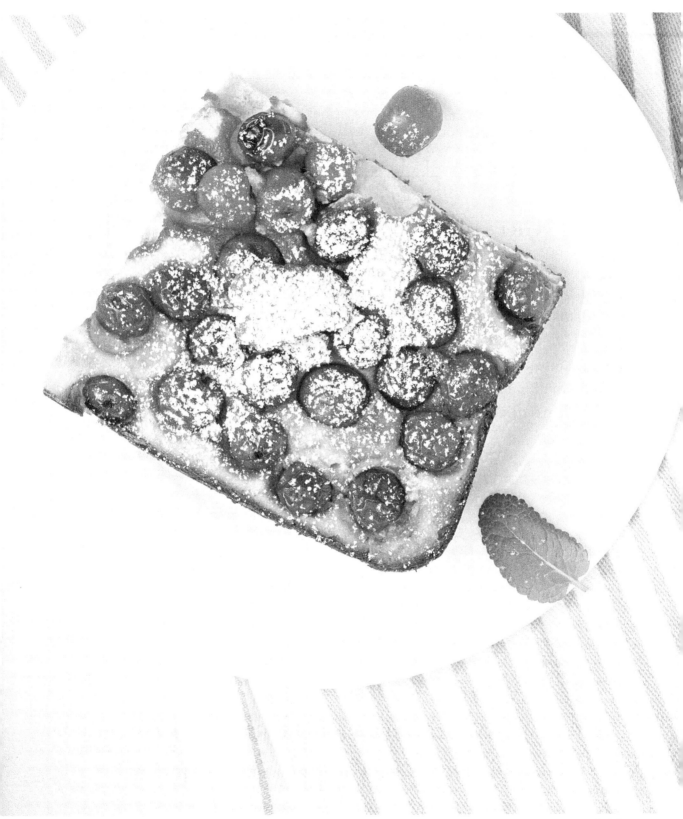

KALE AND ALMONDS

 Cooking Difficulty: 2/10

 Cooking Time: 8 minutes

 Servings: 4

INGREDIENTS

- 1 c. water
- 1 big kale bunch, chopped
- 1 tbsp. balsamic vinegar
- 1/3 c. toasted almonds
- 3 minced garlic cloves
- 1 small chopped yellow onion
- 2 tbsps. olive oil

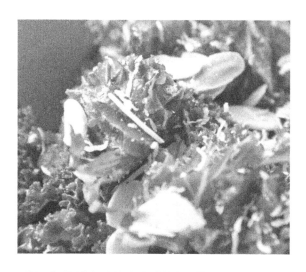

DESCRIPTION

STEP 1
Set your instant pot on sauté mode, add oil, heat it up, add onion, stir and cook for 3 minutes.

STEP 2
Add garlic, water and kale, stir, cover and cook on High for 4 minutes.

STEP 3
Add salt, pepper, vinegar, and almonds, toss well, divide between plates and serve as a side dish.

STEP 4
Enjoy!

NUTRITIONAL INFORMATION
140 Calories, 6g Fat, 1g Carbs, 3g Protein

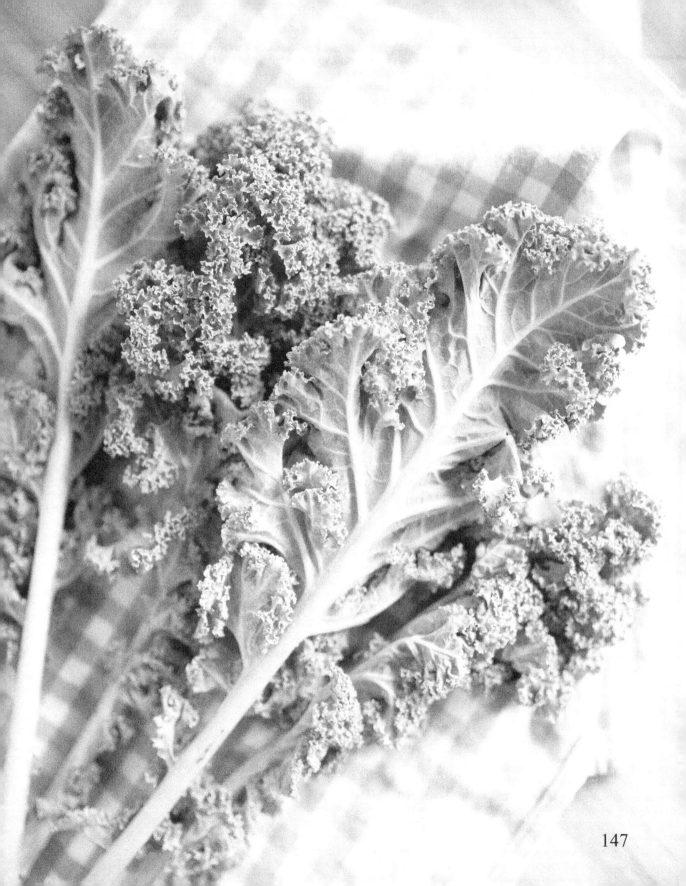

CARROTS WITH THYME AND DILL

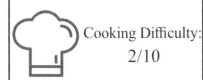 Cooking Difficulty: 2/10	Cooking Time: 7 minutes	Servings: 4

INGREDIENTS

- 1 lb. cubed celery
- 1 c. water
- 2 minced garlic cloves
- salt
- black pepper
- ¼ tsp. dry rosemary
- 1 tbsp. olive oil

DESCRIPTION

STEP 1
Put the water in your instant pot, add steamer basket, add celery cubes inside, cover pot and cook on High for 4 minutes.

STEP 2
In a bowl, mix oil with garlic and rosemary and whisk well.

STEP 3
Add steamed celery, toss well, spread on a lined baking sheet, and introduce in a preheated broiler for 3 minutes. Serve and enjoy as a side dish.

NUTRITIONAL INFORMATION

164 Calories, 10g Fat, 3g Carbs, 3g Protein

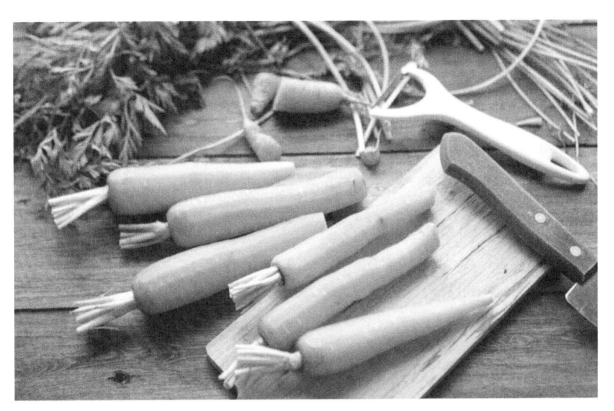

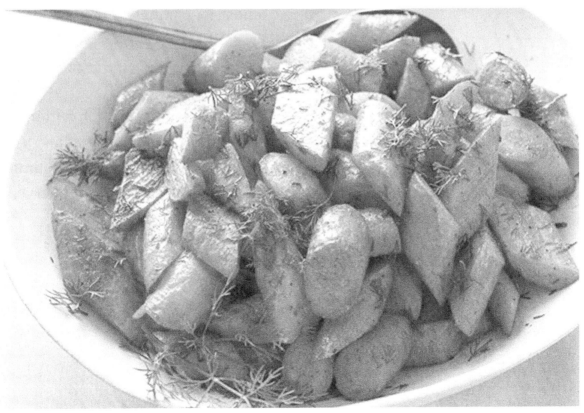

YOGURT MINT

Cooking Difficulty: 2/10	Cooking Time: 5 minutes	Servings: 2

INGREDIENTS

- 1 c. water
- 5 c. vegan milk
- ¾ c. plain yogurt
- ¼ c. fresh mint
- 1 tbsp. maple syrup

DESCRIPTION

STEP 1
Using the Instant Pot Pressure Cooker, add 1 c. water.

STEP 2
Press the Steam function button and adjust to 1 minute. Once done, add the milk.

STEP 3
Press the Yogurt function button and allow to boil. Add in yogurt and fresh mint. Stir well to dissolve. Pour in a glass and add maple syrup. Serve.

NUTRITIONAL INFORMATION
294 Calories, 18g Fat, 6.1g Carbs, 24.2g Protein

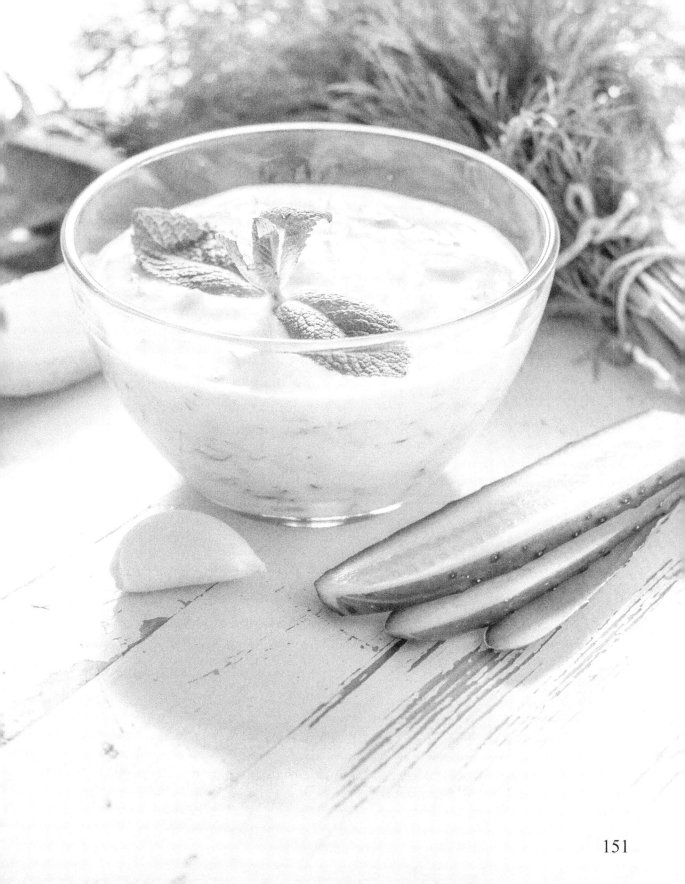

CELERY AND ROSEMARY SIDE DISH

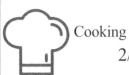 Cooking Difficulty: 2/10	Cooking Time: 8 minutes	Servings: 4

INGREDIENTS

- 1 lb. cubed celery
- 1 c. water
- 2 minced garlic cloves
- salt
- black pepper
- ¼ tsp. dry rosemary
- 1 tbsp. olive oil

DESCRIPTION

STEP 1
Put the water in your instant pot, add steamer basket, add celery cubes inside, cover pot and cook on High for 4 minutes.

STEP 2
In a bowl, mix oil with garlic and rosemary and whisk well.

STEP 3
Add steamed celery, toss well, spread on a lined baking sheet, and introduce in a preheated broiler for 3 minutes. Serve and enjoy as a side dish.

NUTRITIONAL INFORMATION

100 Calories, 13g Fat, 6g Carbs, 3g Protein

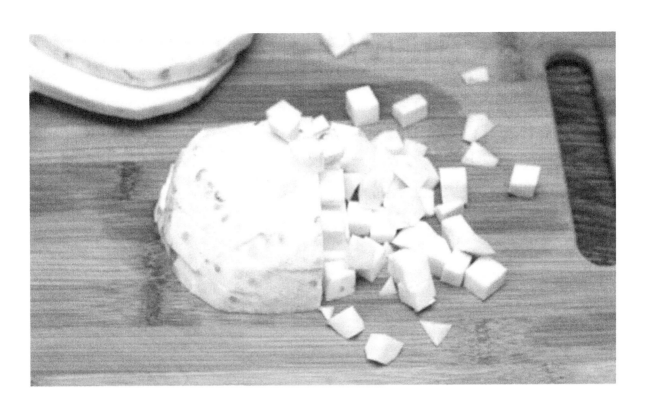

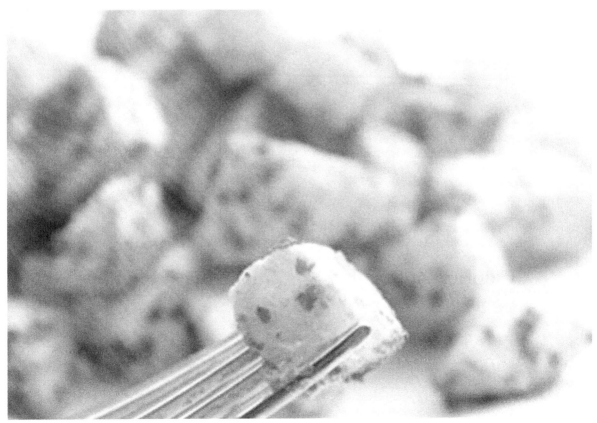

153

CHILI ASPARAGUS

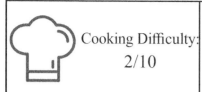 Cooking Difficulty: 2/10	Cooking Time: 128 minutes	Servings: 2

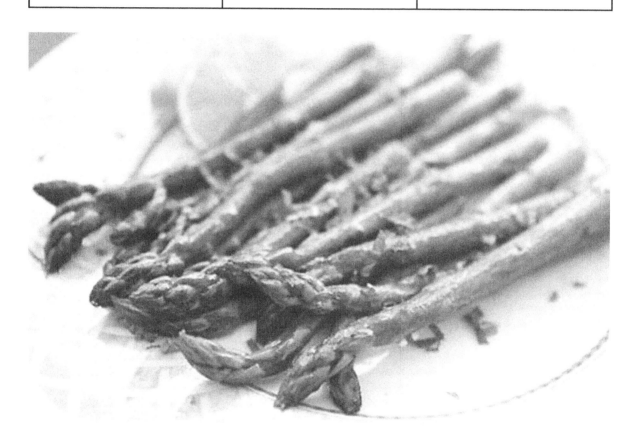

NUTRITIONAL INFORMATION

Calories: 440; Fat: 74g; Carbs: 34g; Protein: 9g

INGREDIENTS

- 1 bundle asparagus
- 1 diced red chili
- ½ tsp. cumin seeds
- 1 tbsp. fresh coriander
- 3 tbsps. olive oil
- ½ of lemon juice
- salt

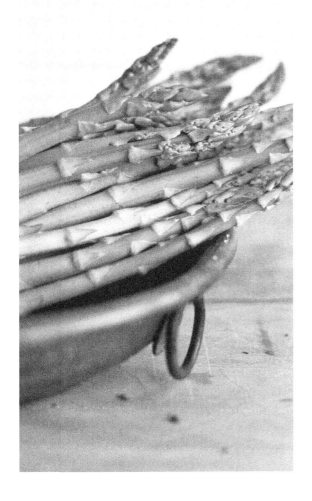

DESCRIPTION

STEP 1
Put together chili, lemon juice, olive oil, cumin, and coriander in a mixing bowl. Mix well.

STEP 2
Transfer the mixture into a cling film and roll. Put inside the refrigerator for 1–2 hours.

STEP 3
Meanwhile, place the asparagus in the Instant Pot Pressure Cooker. Drizzle in olive oil. Close the lid carefully. Press the "slow cook" button and cook for 2 hours.

STEP 4
When the timer beeps, choose the quick pressure release. This would take 1–2 minutes. Remove the lid.

STEP 5
Turn off the pressure cooker. Carefully remove the lid.

STEP 6
Transfer asparagus in a platter. Spread the chili mixture on top of the asparagus. Serve.

NAPA CABBAGE SIDE SALAD

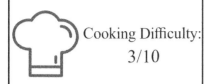 Cooking Difficulty: 3/10

 Cooking Time: 48 minutes

 Servings: 6

INGREDIENTS

- salt
- ground black pepper
- 1 lb. chopped napa cabbage
- 1 carrot, julienned
- 2 tbsps. veggie stock
- ½ c. daikon radish
- 3 minced garlic cloves
- 3 chopped green onion stalks
- 1 tbsp. coconut aminos
- 3 tbsps. chili flakes
- 1 tbsp. olive oil
- ½ inch grated ginger

DESCRIPTION

STEP 1
In a bowl, mix black pepper, cabbage, and salt, massage well for 10 minutes, cover, and leave aside for 30 minutes.

STEP 2
In another bowl, mix chili flakes with aminos, garlic, oil, and ginger, and stir whisk well.

STEP 3
Drain cabbage well, transfer to your instant pot, add the stock, carrots, green onions, radish, and the chili paste you made, stir, cover, and cook on High for 5 minutes. Place on plates and serve!

NUTRITIONAL INFORMATION
103 Calories, 6g Fat, 1g Carbs, 2.2g Protein

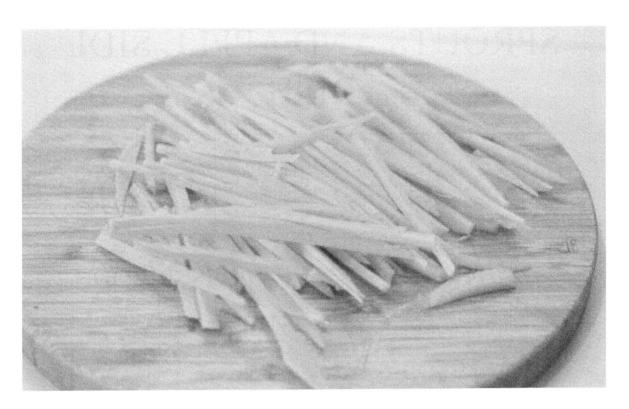

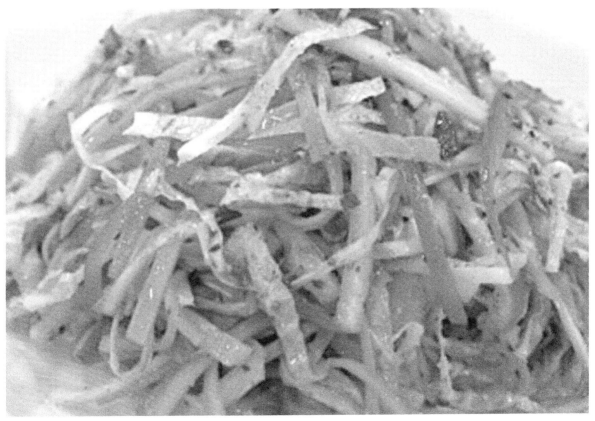

157

SPROUTS AND APPLE SIDE DISH

Cooking Difficulty: 2/10	Cooking Time: 8 minutes	Servings: 4

INGREDIENTS

- 1 julienned green apple
- 1½ tsps. olive oil
- 4 c. alfalfa sprouts
- salt
- black pepper
- ¼ c. coconut milk

DESCRIPTION

STEP 1

Set your instant pot on sauté mode, add oil, heat it up, add apple and sprouts, stir, cover the pot and cook on High for 5 minutes.

STEP 2

Add salt, pepper, and coconut milk, stir, cover the pot again and cook on High for 2 minutes more. Serve and enjoy as a side dish.

NUTRITIONAL INFORMATION

123 Calories, 7g Fat, 2g Carbs, 5g Protein

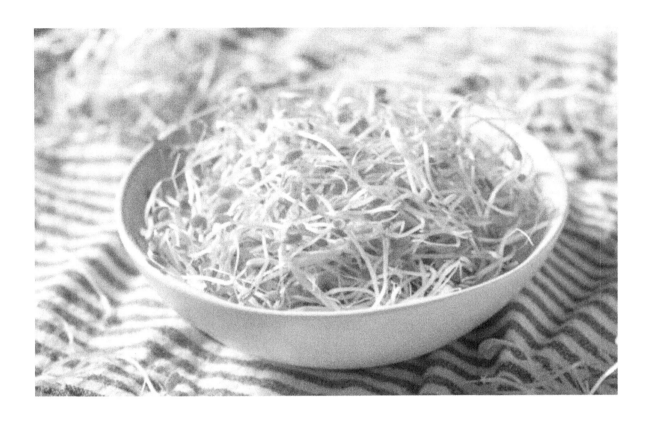

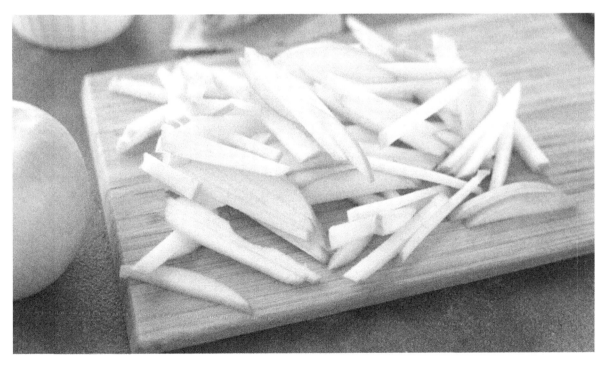

CELERIAC FRIES

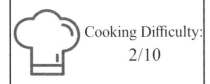 Cooking Difficulty: 2/10	Cooking Time: 9 minutes	Servings: 2

INGREDIENTS

- 2 big peeled celeriac
- 1 c. water
- salt
- ¼ tsp. baking soda
- olive oil

DESCRIPTION

STEP 1
Put the water in your instant pot, add salt and the baking soda and the steamer basket, add celeriac fries inside, cover, cook on High for 4 minutes, drain and transfer them to a bowl.

STEP 2
Place olive oil on a pan and heat over medium-high heat, add celeriac fries, cook until they are golden on all sides, drain grease, transfer them to plates and serve as a side dish.

STEP 3
Enjoy!

NUTRITIONAL INFORMATION

194 Calories, 9g Fat, 3g Carbs, 3g Protein

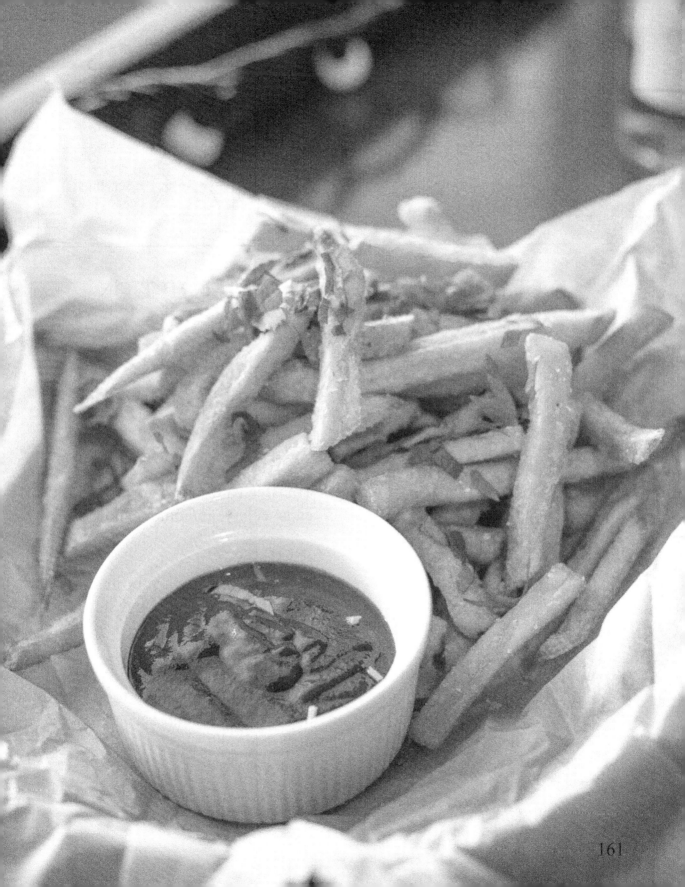

CAULIFLOWER AND EGGS SALAD

 Cooking Difficulty: 2/10	Cooking Time: 7 minutes	Servings: 10

INGREDIENTS

- 21 oz. cauliflower, separate the florets
- 1 c. chopped red onion
- 1 c. chopped celery
- ½ c. water
- salt
- black pepper
- 2 tbsps. balsamic vinegar
- 1 tsp. stevia
- 4 boiled and chopped eggs
- 1 c. mayonnaise

DESCRIPTION

STEP 1
Put the water in your instant pot, add steamer basket, add cauliflower, cover pot, and cook on High for 5 minutes.

STEP 2
Transfer cauliflower to a bowl, add eggs, celery, and onion, and toss.

STEP 3
In a separate bowl, mix mayo with salt, pepper, vinegar, and stevia and whisk well.

STEP 4
Add this to your salad, toss, divide between plates and serve as a side dish. Enjoy!

NUTRITIONAL INFORMATION

171 Calories, 9g Fat, 2g Carbs, 5g Protein

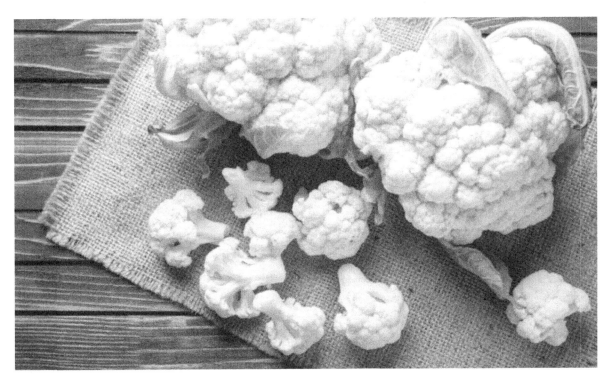

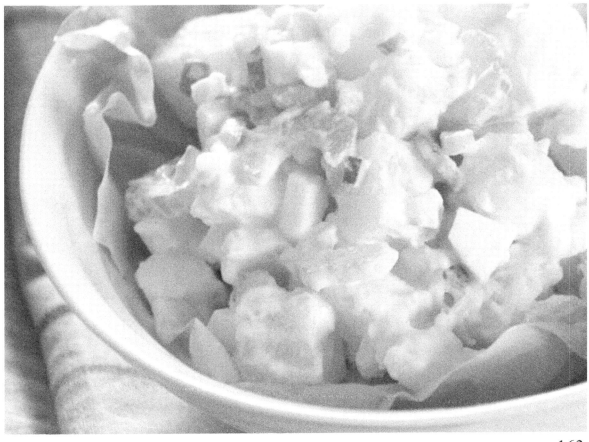

RASPBERRY COMPOTE

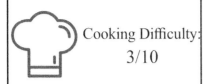 Cooking Difficulty: 3/10	Cooking Time: 27 minutes	Servings: 4

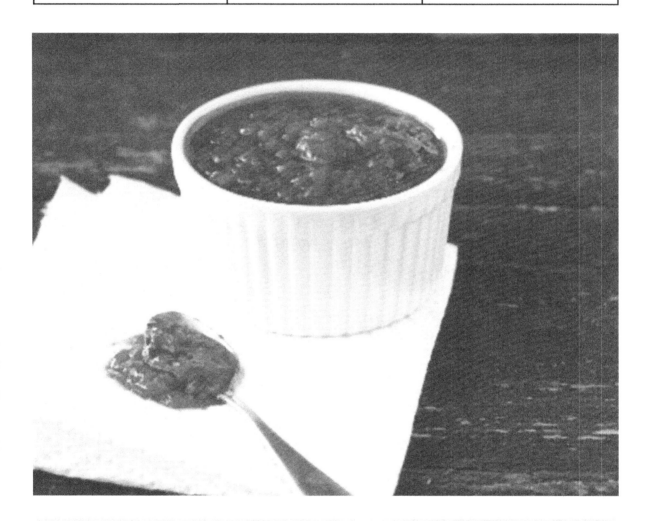

NUTRITIONAL INFORMATION

148 Calories, 6.9g Fat, 1.7g Carbs, 3.5g Protein

INGREDIENTS

- 2 c. raspberries
- 1 c. swerve
- 1 tsp. grated orange zest
- 1 tsp. vanilla

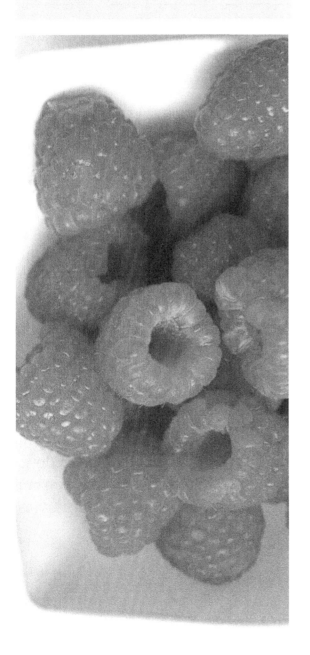

DESCRIPTION

STEP 1
Plug in your instant pot and press the 'Saute' button. Add raspberries, swerve, orange zest, and vanilla extract. Stir well and pour in 1 cup of water. Cook for 5 minutes, stirring constantly.

STEP 2
Now pour in 2 more cups of water and press the 'Cancel' button. Seal the lid and set the steam release handle to the 'Sealing' position. Press the 'Manual' button and set the timer for 15 minutes on low pressure.

STEP 3
When you hear the cooker's end signal, press the 'Cancel' button and release the pressure naturally for 10-15 minutes. Move the pressure handle to the 'Venting' position to release any remaining pressure and open the lid.

STEP 4
Optionally, stir some more lemon juice and transfer to serving bowls.

STEP 5
Chill to a room temperature and refrigerate for one hour before serving.

PUMPKIN PIE PANCAKES

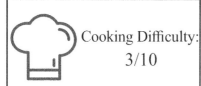 Cooking Difficulty: 3/10	Cooking Time: 23 minutes	Servings: 4

INGREDIENTS

- 1 c. pumpkin puree
- 3 large eggs
- 2 tbsps. swerve
- ¾ c. almond flour
- 4 tbsps. unsweetened almond milk
- 1 tsp. pumpkin pie seasoning
- ¼ tsp. salt
- 2 tbsps. baking powder

DESCRIPTION

STEP 1

In a mixing bowl, mix pumpkin pie seasoning, eggs, swerve, and almond milk. With a whisking attachment on, beat well on high speed. Gradually add flour, salt, baking powder, and pumpkin pie seasoning. Continue to mix for another 2 minutes. Finally, add the pumpkin puree and mix well again.

STEP 2

Plugin your instant pot and press the 'Saute' button. Grease the stainless steel insert with some oil and heat up. Add about ¼ cup of the batter and cook for 3 minutes. When done, gently remove from your instant pot and top with some blueberries, raspberries, or almonds.

NUTRITIONAL INFORMATION

143 Calories, 10g Fat, 3.7g Carbs, 5.9g Protein

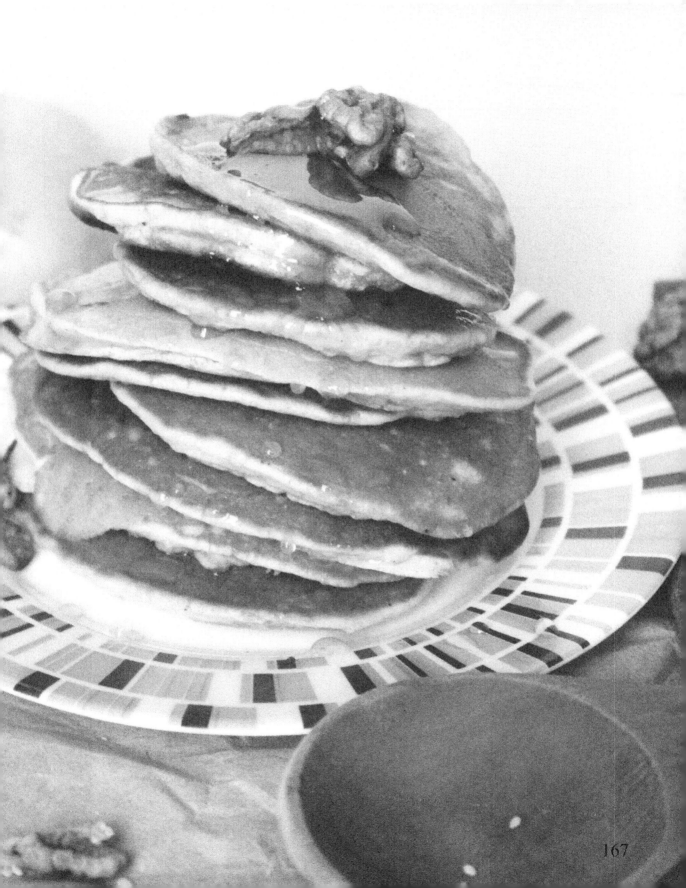

CACAO AVOCADO CAKE

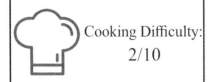 Cooking Difficulty: 2/10	Cooking Time: 23 minutes	Servings: 3

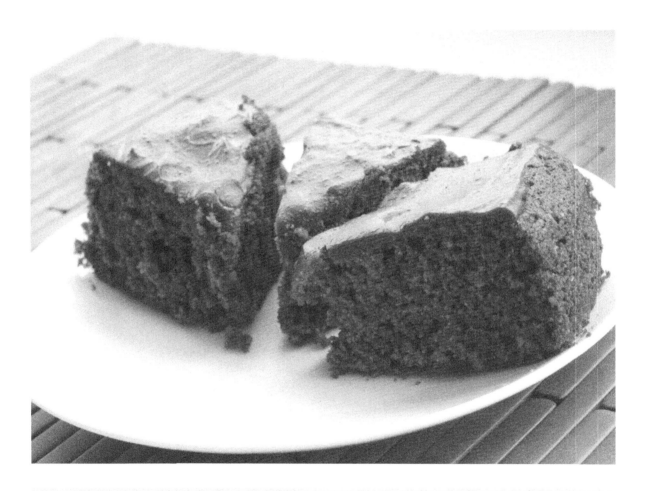

NUTRITIONAL INFORMATION

349.7 Calories, 30.9g Fat, 11.7g Carbs, 3.5g Protein

INGREDIENTS

- ¼ c. avocado, mashed
- 1 ripe banana
- ½ c. cocoa powder
- ½ tsp. apple cider vinegar
- 3 tbsps. coconut oil, melted
- 2 tbsps. sweetener (your choice)
- ¾ tsp. baking soda
- 2 tsps. fresh lemon juice
- 1 c. water

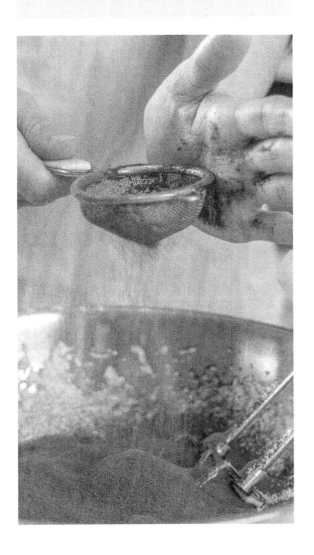

DESCRIPTION

STEP 1
Blend all ingredients in a blender.

STEP 2
Lightly grease three mini ramekins with coconut oil. Pour the batter into ramekins until they are about 3 of the way full.

STEP 3
Pour the water into your Instant Pot and add the steaming rack. Place the pans onto the steaming rack.

STEP 4
Close and lock the lid. Press MANUAL for high pressure and set the cooking time to 18 minutes.

STEP 5
Use the quick release of the pressure by flipping the valve on the lid.

STEP 6
Serve warm or cold.

RICE PUDDING

Cooking Difficulty: 2/10	Cooking Time: 13 minutes	Servings: 2

INGREDIENTS

- ½ c. short grain rice
- 1 cinnamon stick
- 1 ½ c. vegan milk
- 1 slice lemon peel
- salt
- 2 tbsps. sweetener (your choice)

DESCRIPTION

STEP 1
Rinse the rice under cold water. Using the Instant Pot Pressure Cooker, put the milk, cinnamon stick, sweetener, salt, and lemon peel inside.

STEP 2
Close the lid. Lock in place and make sure to seal the valve. Press the "pressure" button and cook for 10 minutes on high.

STEP 3
When the timer beeps, choose the quick pressure release. This would take 1–2 minutes. Remove the lid. Open the pressure cooker and discard the lemon peel and cinnamon stick. Spoon in a serving bowl and serve.

NUTRITIONAL INFORMATION

Calories: 111, Fat: 1.6g, Carbs: 21g, Protein: 3.3g

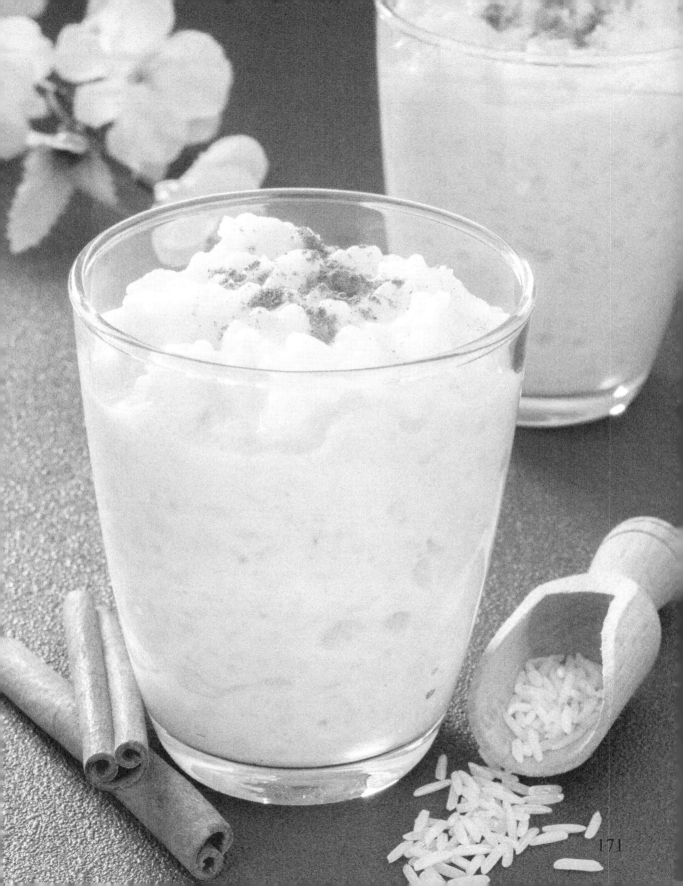

VANILLA CREAM

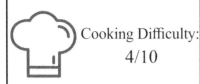

Cooking Difficulty:
4/10

Cooking Time:
28 minutes

Servings:
4

INGREDIENTS

- 8 large eggs
- ¾ c. unsweetened almond milk
- 1½ c. heavy cream

- 1 tsp. vanilla extract, sliced and seeded
- 1 vanilla bean
- 4 tbsps. swerve

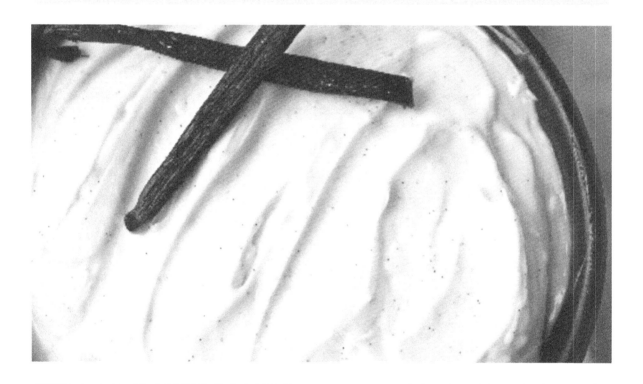

NUTRITIONAL INFORMATION

309 Calories, 27.3g Fat, 2.3g Carbs, 13.7g Protein

DESCRIPTION

STEP 1
Place vanilla extract in a mixing bowl along with the remaining ingredients.

STEP 2
With a whisking attachment on, beat the mixture for 2 minutes on high speed and transfer into 4 ramekins. Tightly wrap with aluminum foil and set aside.

STEP 3
Plug in your instant pot and pour in 2 cups of water. Set the trivet at the bottom of the stainless steel insert and carefully place the ramekins on top.

STEP 4
Seal the lid and set the steam release handle to the 'Sealing' position. Press the 'Manual' button and set the timer for 15 minutes.

STEP 5
When done, perform a quick release by moving the pressure valve to the 'Venting' position.

STEP 6
Open the lid and carefully remove the ramekins from your instant pot.

STEP 7
Cool to room temperature without removing the aluminum foil.

STEP 8
Transfer to the fridge and cool completely before serving.

CHERRY PUDDING

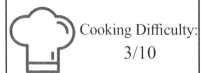 Cooking Difficulty: 3/10	Cooking Time: 11 minutes	Servings: 5

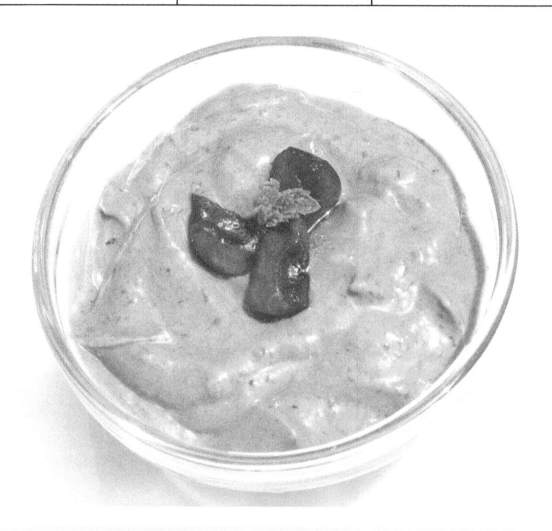

NUTRITIONAL INFORMATION

153 Calories, 14g Fat, 2g Carbs, 4.5g Protein

INGREDIENTS

- ¾ c. whipped cream
- ¾ c. unsweetened almond milk
- 4 egg whites
- 3 tsps. powdered stevia
- 1 tsp. sugar-free cherry extract
- ¼ tsp. xanthan gum

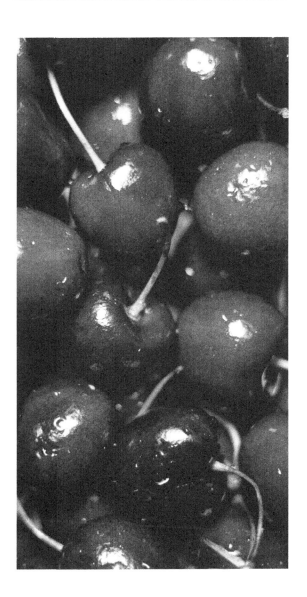

DESCRIPTION

STEP 1

In a mixing bowl, mix almond milk, heavy cream, and egg whites. Beat well on high, for 3 minutes. Pour the mixture into 5 ramekins.

STEP 2

Plug in your instant pot and pour 2 cups of water into the stainless steel insert. Position a trivet at the bottom and place the ramekins on top. Securely lock the lid and adjust the steam release handle. Press the "Manual" button and set the timer for 3 minutes. Cook on high pressure.

STEP 3

When you hear the cooker's end signal, press the "Cancel" button and release the pressure naturally.

STEP 4

Open the pot and chill the pudding to room temperature. Refrigerate for 1 hour before serving.

CONCLUSION

I sincerely hope that you have enjoyed reading this recipe book as much as I have enjoyed writing it. I am confident that my recipe collection will offer you some new and healthy options to add to your daily diet. The best thing that I discovered while writing this book is that your meals do not have to be tasteless and boring to be healthy. I wish you immense success in adding new and healthier meal choices to your diet—that is not only good for you but taste delightful!

Henry Irving

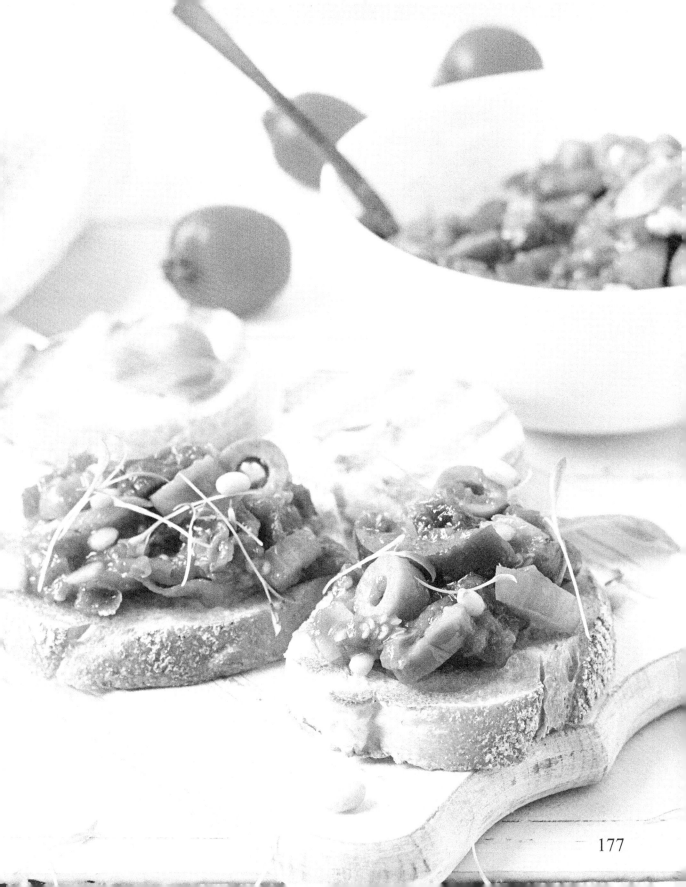

Made in the USA
Monee, IL
15 December 2022

21759873R00098